1

CHIA FOR HEALTH

By Gloria J. Hoover

ISBN 978-0-6152-3845-6

This book is intended as an educational and informational resource, and for reference only. The information is designed to make you better informed about the subject. If you have a medical or nutritional problem or question, please seek the care of a doctor or other trained professional. The publisher and author expressly disclaim any responsibility or liability in connection with the use of this book.

Dedication

This book is dedicated to all the men and women that work so hard to bring chia to us, from the researchers, the growers, the mills and the promoters of the seeds. This is a wonderful food product and without the numerous people working we would not know about the new super power food of the future.

TABLE OF CONTENTS

Chia for Health

Our Journey

My husband and I were in a bookstore just looking around at what might be interesting, something different, just browsing the store. All of a sudden, there on the spine of a book was the word CHIA. Chia, you mean like in chia pets at Holiday time? So down that book came, as we leafed through the pages, sections about health, diabetes, omega-3's, and other areas caught our eye. Needless to say that book went home with us and that was the start of our long journey researching and using chia seeds.

This was late in 2001 or early 2002 and not much information was available about chia. The web searches told a little about omega-3 essential fatty acid as they related to flax and fish oils. Then the search for chia seeds begins with the local health food stores. Talk about strange looks! The store help would always ask "you mean like chia pets", "never heard of people eating the seeds", "are you sure it is safe". Those were just a few of the responses. Heedless to say, we didn't find any chia seeds locally. Thank goodness for the internet and web searches. Then the second surprise only two places sold chia seeds!

Our first order was placed and arrived the day before we were leaving on a business trip, family wedding and vacation to Los Angles, California. My husband's younger sister was getting married to her high school sweetheart with my husband giving the Bride away meaning we were involved in rehearsals and affairs of the wedding. Los Angles was in the middle of July 4th celebrations and a heat wave. We had driven down from the Seattle, Washington area with our big pickup truck.

The first stop was to pick up bottled water for the business trip portion of selecting merchandise at one of our suppliers. We knew it was going to take several hours of roaming around a big open warehouse that wasn't air conditioned! Yep, it was hot, humid and really tiring.

Mission accomplished and off to the hotel near the family. Once settled in, had our afternoon portion of chia and then off to dinner with the family. Have I mentioned how hot it was and how heat just seems to sap the energy, making you feel tired, sleepy? Later that night, we're back at the hotel watching TV. One of us said – are you tired? No was the answer. This is strange, it is hours after our normal bed time and here we are watching TV. At this point the phone rings, it is the bride wanting us to meet them for breakfast at 7 AM.

That breakfast was just the start of a long, hot, busy day. Last minute hurrying, lunch with the family, sitting around talking, more errands to run. Oh, you know the typical wedding stuff. That evening was dinner with the wedding party; I went back to the hotel to do some computer work, husband to the rehearsal. On his return the conversation was similar to the night before – are you tired? No, well this is strange it must be the excitement. Or just maybe it is the chia??

Wedding day, the bride is beautiful, the groom handsome and after a few bumps and misplaced items it is off to the reception high on a hill. Did I mention the heat wave that was occurring? It was so hot, so humid, yet we were full of energy. Ah, it must be the excitement once again. After kisses and hugs, off we start back to Seattle on this hot Sunday night of that 4th of July weekend.

We crossed over the Grapevine into Bakersfield and saw traffic, traffic as far as you could see. Bumper to bumper slow moving traffic inching the way up the central valley. Is there an accident? Nope this was just the Holiday traffic back to San Francisco! Hundreds of miles, crawling, running out of CD's, and still the lines of traffic snake slowly up the valley. We stopped a few times as it was getting late, no room at the Inn we were told, and on we went long into the night.

At last a hotel room, it was the last one! It is now around 11PM and we should be tired or even better sound asleep. Yet once again, we were watching TV, laughing and talking. Could it really be the chia??

During the next few months we stopped using chia, then would start again and each time would notice that we felt better, were less tired, had more energy. I noticed my skin was softer, smoother. Husband noticed that the winkles around my eyes (crow's feet to most of us) were going away. The nails were a little stronger and the hair was getting shiner. The only thing we were doing differently was using chia every day.

Over the course of the next few years, we researched as much as we could about chia, omega-3's, and the vitamins and minerals contained in chia.

This book is the accumulation of that research.

IN THE BEGINNING

Evidence has been discovered that chia may have been used at food as early as 1500 BC in what is known today as central Mexico. At that time, chia was mainly used by itself, mixed with other grains or seeds, or mixed with water for a refreshing drink or ground into flour. Chia was also used as a medicine, pressed for the oil and even used as a base for body and face paints.

At one time chia was a generic or broad based term used to describe a variety of plants in the region of Mesoamerica (Mexico) and the American Southwest. These plants grew wild and all chia plants are a member of the cosmopolitan mint family, Lamiaceae. There are a number of species of Chia that are grown in the American Southwest (California and Arizona mainly), the high plateaus of Mexico thru Central America, Peru and Bolivia in South America. Chia plants thrive in deep sandy clay soils. Today, much of Chia grown in other locations is used for different purposes than food. Until recently many of the artisans in Mexico used the oil from the lower grades of chia as a finish on their hand painted pottery. Chia oil was superior to other oils as it added a higher gloss and was more resisted to wear.

Today some lower grades of chia seeds are made into animal feed. Just as the seeds and oil are nutritious to humans, the seeds and oil are equal good for our animals.

The species of Chia that is high in omega-3, vitamins and minerals is known by the Latin name Salvia hispanica L. (the L. means Latin name). Salvia hispanica is an annual herb with grains/seeds that are small, oval and brown/black with reddish brown markings. Fully matured Chia has a lack of color or pigment causing the grains to appear white. Chiatic is the Aztec root word of chia used to describe something with an oil or greasy substance. When ground the chia flour is very oily/greasy because of the omega-3 oils.

Chia naturally repels both insects and other plants. Grazing animals such as cattle and deer do not consider chia plants to be a tasty snack and will avoid the area where the plants are growing. Most of the current information reports that chia is the forgotten food of the Aztecs yet chia was a major food crop years long before the Aztec rise to power. The Teotihuacan civilization was between 100 B.C. to around 850 A. D. with very advanced agriculture practices. Because of these techniques, the Teotihuacan produced enough food to support the 200,000 people that lived in the central city. This technology included massive irrigation projects and terracing of the land.

After the fall of Teotihuacan, the Toltecs came into power and quickly expanded their influence over what is now central Mexico. While in power until around 1165 A.D, the Toltecs expanded and build upon agriculture techniques used prior to their conquest and ruled with authority until the Aztecs, also called Mexicas, came down into the area from a place to the north called Aztlan. The exact location of Aztlan has never been located. The Aztec civilization was at its greatest power between 1168 and 1521 until the Spanish conquerors invaded the New World.

According to several historical documents from the Toltec period, chia was an important source of food and was even used as a type of currency to pay what we might consider taxes.

The Aztecs learned the farming technique from the Toltecs of reclaiming marsh lands by weaving nets with vines and soil to form islands. These islands then where used to produce food and chia was grown on some of the islands.

Chia was so important, considered so valuable that the first Aztec rulers limited the grain to only the people of the royal court including the Doctors and other staff members. As time went on, the servants or slaves of the court noticed the health of people of the court and started smuggling the grain out to their family members. Within a relatively short time span chia was a staple food, used as medicine and for political and religious ceremonies. Now most of us know about the bloody thirsty rituals of the Aztecs so we won't go into any detail about those! Chia was used more as a symbol of the power of the Gods. The seeds were ground and made into a paste that was formed into the shape of a particular God then eaten to empower the people with those attributes.

Archaeologists have also discovered containers of chia buried with the Aztec emperors much like food is found in the tombs of Egypt.

Both chia and flax seeds both contain large amounts of triglyceride and are rich in linolenic fatty acid, we call that fatty acid omega-3 oil. Flax has antinutritional cyanogenic glucosides that react badly with vitamin B6 and flax is also very hard to digest. The Aztec people were aware of flax as it is mentioned in several documents yet was never used as a food source. Chia, on the other hand, was revered, used by the warriors for energy and endurance and was a major food source equaled to only maize and amaranth.

When Cortez and his men landed in the Aztec empire, the civilization was flourishing; cities were huge compared to the European settlements. What is now Mexico City was called Tenochtitlan and had a population of roughly 200,000 people. Tenochtitlan was twice the size of the either London or Rome, with a marketplace filled with exotic foods, staples, and a tremendous variety of products.

Just the size of one city square was larger than most Spanish cities. Most of the homes had large plots of land that grew chia as well as other staple foods of that time. According to letters, scrolls, and codex from religious leaders, soldiers and others the Aztec cities and land were marvels; the culture had a complex religion, a strong army, commerce and a huge knowledge of botany for both food and health purposes.

History has taught about the fall of the Aztec civilization to the Spanish conquerors. Along with the conquest, there were food shortages causes by natural disasters such as droughts and possibly earthquakes. One thing that the Spanish were quite good at was breaking apart the people and rebuilding their conquered lands. One of the first things to occur was to destroy the religion and that included chia. The Spanish didn't understand what an important food source chia was but did understand the religious purposes so in their own way banned chia.

Chia was then only grown on small family plots away from the major areas of the country. As the years past, chia was forgotten, used more as a refreshing beverage on a hot day.

Chia was also a main dietary staple of the Mayans not just the Azetcs. In fact, the Mexican State of Chiapas, which was located in Mayan territory, gets its name from the Nahuatl word Chiapan which mean "river of chia". Fortunately during the last 30 years, a few people including Ricardo Ayerza JR. and Wayne Coates have developed new techniques, new research and are reviving this ancient food for our modern day lives.

What Makes Chia Special?

Chia is packed full of wonderful vitamins and minerals that our bodies need to maintain our health, energy and mental clarity. Much of the current suggestions for chia are for omega-3 and fiber but did you know that it also is a great source of protein? Fasten those seat belts as here we go!

Difference between Chia Seed and Chia Oil

When shopping for chia you will find chia seed, chia oil and capsules of chia oil. So what is the difference? Basically the only difference between the seeds and oil is that the oil does not contain any fiber. Most of the chia oil is cold pressed from the seeds. While there are other methods that can be used to extract the oil please only purchase cold pressed – this method is similar to that used to extract olive oil – and does not heat the oil. Heating chia oil will cause it to oxide and that is not a good thing! That said chia oil should not be used in cooking such as sautéing or frying. Chia oil is wonderful used in salad dressings, smoothies, or drizzled over other foods. The other main difference between chia oil and the gel capsules is the oil is considered to be a food product while the gel capsules are considered to a dietary supplement.

Why would I want to purchase the oil instead of the capsules if the oil is the same oil? Some people cannot tolerant taking capsules, while others are vegan and the capsules themselves contain gelatin. Another reason may totally surprise you. Chia oil is wonderful for the skin! Some people even use a small amount on their hair and scalp. Remember all those omega-3's in chia? Chia oil absorbs into the skin very quickly, hydrating the cells and taking with the oil all the wonderful vitamins and minerals into those cells. But more about that a little later in the skin care section.

To summarize if you want extra fiber in your diet you should choose the seeds, if you want the food product use the seeds but if you are looking for a dietary supplement then purchase the capsules or oil.

BORDERS.

BORDERS
BOOKS MUSIC AND CAFE
30 Square Drive
Victor, NY 14564
(585) 421-9230

STORE: 0364   REG: 02/59   TRAN#: 6466
SALE   01/14/2009   EMP: 01930

CHIA FOR HEALTH
                        ST T   19.95
Order#:63228

                Subtotal   19.95
                NEW YORK 7.125%   1.42
1   Item   Total   21.37
                CASH   25.37
                Cash Change Due   4.00

01/14/2009 03:31PM

card.

Exchanges of opened audio books, music, videos, video games, software and electronics will be permitted subject to the same time periods and receipt requirements as above and can be made for the same item only.

Periodicals, newspapers, comic books, food and drink, digital downloads, gift cards, return gift cards, items marked "non-returnable," "final sale" or the like and out-of-print, collectible or pre-owned items cannot be returned or exchanged.

Returns and exchanges to a Borders, Borders Express or Waldenbooks retail store of merchandise purchased from Borders.com may be permitted in certain circumstances. See Borders.com for details.

BORDERS®

Returns

Returns of merchandise purchased from a Borders, Borders Express or Waldenbooks retail store will be permitted only if presented in saleable condition accompanied by the original sales receipt or Borders gift receipt within the time periods specified below. Returns accompanied by the original sales receipt must be made within 30 days of purchase and the purchase price will be refunded in the same form as the original purchase. Returns accompanied by the original Borders gift receipt must be made within 60 days of purchase and the purchase price will be refunded in the form of a return gift card.

Exchanges of opened audio books, music, videos, video games, software and electronics will be permitted subject to the same time periods and receipt requirements as above and can be made for the same item only.

Periodicals, newspapers, comic books, food and drink, digital downloads, gift cards, return gift cards, items marked "non-returnable," "final sale" or the like and out-of-print, collectible or pre-owned items cannot be returned or exchanged.

Grade or Quality of Chia Seeds

Just a few short years ago there were only two main areas that produced chia seeds – Argentina and Mexico. Peru started producing chia in more "modern" times. Some chia is grown in the American Southwest just not on a large commercial scale. Other countries do grow chia and most of it is not for human use yet it used in other products as the omega3 and other nutrients are very low. Within the last few years chia grown in new locations are starting to appear in the market. We suggest that you look at these seeds with caution because the demand for chia is sky rocketing some of the new locations are producing chia seeds in mass but when tested the seeds are low quality and some not cleaned well (pieces of seed hulls and other plant materials are packaged in the bag). Much of the time you will see packages that say highest grade, 60% omega-3 and those are the seeds to purchase. If the price seems to be much lower than other companies, the seeds look strange or even have an off or bitter taste switch to a little more expensive brand of chia. Remember that old saying of you get what you pay for. Still not sure about your seeds? Ask the store, web site or seller where the seeds or oils are grown, are they cleaned, and what percentage is the omega-3 (the name that might appear on the certificate of analysis is Alpha Linolenic Acid).

Not all chia seeds are equal in nutrients and not all chia being sold is of the highest quality or agricultural standards. Remember those Chia Pets please do not eat those seed! They are not meant for eating but to be used for the chia pets. Many times the seeds are very low quality, unknown sources and many have been treated with pesticides.

We have also started seeing all sorts of "interesting" claims on web sites that our chia is the best, our chia is white chia that is ground and that means you get more nutrients. I am sure you have seen those same or similar statements being made. So what is the truth?

All most all the chia on the market is from Peru (the white chia), Mexico or Argentina with all the test results showing about 1 percent difference in some of the nutrients and that is a very small difference. Chia does not need to be ground and will lose some of the omega-3 oil if ground. Personally I want the whole seed with all the oil intact. We feel that grinding the seed, then packaging it you would have to lose some of the nutrients just as you would in any fruit or vegetable that is sliced, ground or processed. Recently there are reports of toasted ground chia seed being marketed and that it is so much more nutritious. Since the seeds have been ground, the omega-3 is lost, and the toasting can removed some of the vitamins and minerals. Why would it be more nutritious? If you take one tablespoon of chia seeds and match it to one tablespoon of the powder you would appear to have more volume. It is suggested that you asked the company for their lab reports to verify any claims before making your purchase.

The best way to purchase chia is the whole seed, the mixed colors and the current crop. If for some reason, the seeds are not right for your diet then the cold pressed oil or soft gel caps is the best option.

As of this writing there is no certified organic chia so do not be mis-lead by some of the web sites and packaging. Chia is naturally organic as was stated earlier. Certified organic means that the government has inspected the processing, transportation, and storage facilities and it all complies with the current laws for organic. If your bag doesn't have that USDA certified organic seal, it is not certified. Sometime mid-2008 a limited quality of USDA certified organic chia seed will be available on the market with more to be grown and processed.

Chia versus Fish Oil

Remember the old cod liver oil back in our younger years? I am sure some of us that are a little older remember that smell, the awful taste and the lecture from Mom about how good is was for us. Fast forward to now, it isn't call cod liver oil today but fish oil. Fish oil that has been processed so it has no fishy odor or taste and the source of the fish isn't mentioned. I'm one of those that break out in hives if I come in contact with mercury so have to be very careful of which fish I eat and how often. That means I want to know where my fish oil is from, what type of fish, etc. To add to the fish oil problem, farmed raised fish lack the omega-3 of wild caught fish.

Why worry about fish oil when there is chia seed or oil! Chia contains the same type of ALA and converts it to EPA and DHA which have the same benefits as fish oil but without the smell or taste, or toxic substances that can be found in fish. Chia does not contain cholesterol as does most fish oils. Unlike fish oil, Chia's omega-3 is balanced to the omega-6. Fish oil is often poorly regulated and can vary in the quality. There are many different types of fish allergies but chia has not known allergic reactions. Fish oil can be partially hydrogenated which means those nasty trans-fats that we should not ingest while chia contains zero trans-fats. Fish are not a renewable source while chia is a plant that is harvested without hurting the environment.

Fish oil can cause diarrhea, belching, bloating and flatulence (gas). Chia is easy to digest and has the needed fiber for the intestine and digestive tract.

Caution should be used by people with either diabetes or schizophrenia as they may lack the ability to convert ALA to EPA and DHA. This means they should get their omega-3 by either fish oil, chia seed or chia oil. Fish oils can also elevate fasting blood sugar levels. Chia seed or oil doesn't have these properties.

It is important to stress pregnant women, nursing mothers, young children and women who might become pregnant should not eat several species of fish or their fish oils. These fish include swordfish, salmon, herring, tuna, shark and mackerel. All of these fish can contain mercury and other containments.

Chia versus Flax

Chia and flax are both plant seeds / grains and both contain many of the same vitamins and minerals. So why use chia instead of flax?

High quality chia contains between 60 to 65 percent omega-3 oil while high quality flax contains about 53 to 58 percent.

Chia contains a much higher level of antioxidants, more fiber, more protein and more vitamins, and more calcium than flax.

Flax can be genetically modified (GMO) and more GMO flax is currently being grown. During the time this book was published there is no GMO chia being grown and there are no plans for that type of chia to be grown.

Flax must be ground prior to use and must be keep cold after grinding and used in a short time period or the oils contained will go rancid. Flax seed oil has a "strange" taste for many people, must be kept refrigerated, and has a very short shelf life.

Flax is also a main compound of linseed oil, which is the stuff used in the paint industry.

Chia is shelf stable with a reported shelf life of over 2 years, can be stored in a dry room temperature location, does not needed to be ground or processed before using, and is easy to digest.

Flax contains phytostrogens and phytosterols that are hard for many people to digest and interferes with B6.

Children generally do not tolerant flax they do not like the taste or the texture and it is hard for them to digest. Most children like the taste and texture of chia and it is easy for all ages to digest. Kids also like the chia that is mixed with water and has turned to the gel state. Kids really like the taste of chia versus fish oil!

What is Omega-3?

There are three major types of omega-3 essential fatty acids used by the body: Alpha Linolenic Acid (ALA), eicosapentaenoic acid (EPA) and docosahexaenoic acid (DHA). When a food that contains the right type of ALA is eaten, the body converts the ALA to EPA and DHA. The human body does not convert foods into essential fat acids such as omega-3 but must receive them from the foods we eat.

Essential fatty acids or EFA's where once called vitamin F and their metabolites perform two vital body functions. First, they are used to produce the structural part of the membrane barrier that surrounds cells and organelles or intracellular factories. The other function is the passing of information between cells or what is known as signaling.

Research studies done in 2004 suggested that even the healthiest diet is lacking in essential fatty acids leading into all sorts of health problems including heart disease, the nervous system, a host of neurological disorders, learning and behavioral problems, and even memory problems, some types of cancer, depression, inflammation in the body and more problems that had been thought to be unrelated yet appear to be related to the lack of essential fatty acids in the diet. It has also been found that if essential fatty acids are so important to brain active then they must play a role in neurodevelopment disorders including ADHD (attention deficit hyperactivity disorder) and even dyslexia.

Researchers at Purdue University in West Lafayette, Indiana discovered that children with ADHD have lower levels of essential fatty acids, display symptoms of EFA deficiency, and if those lower levels of essential fatty acids include omega-3, had more learning problems, more temper tantrums and other behavior problems plus more health problems.

Further research that included increasing the essential fatty acids in the proper ratio of about 1:1 to around 4:1 of omega-3 to omega-6, the children became calmer, less behavioral problems, slightly better health and would sleep better.

When researchers first discovered these fatty acids, they named them essential as they are essential to normal growth in children and animals. Even a small amount of omega-3 will enable a normal growth, mental activity and nervous system enhancement.

Omega-6 was found to be better at supporting dermal integrity and renal functions leading researchers, at that time, to concentrate their research on omega-6 vs. omega-3.

Only in the last several decades have researchers looked at omega-3 and this has lead to much expanded research with m findings being published almost month'

While the research continu'
diseases seem to stem fror
diet, the major finding ;
consuming more ome
omega-6.

Current researche'
the best ratio she
should be somewh

omega-3 to omega-6. Omega-6 abounds in the Western diet and is found in corn products. Does this mean we should just not eat corn? No, we still need omega-6 from corn and other products. The sad part is that corn products are hidden in all sorts of food – from malt vinegar to caramel color to high fructose syrups that are in so many foods and drinks. Since it is virtually impossible to control all the intake of omega-6 we need to increase the consummation of omega-3.

Research continues into the impact of omega-3 on many diseases and disorders. Some of the newer research is showing the anti-inflammatory components are even having an effect on some heart diseases and may prove more effective than just lowering the bad cholesterol alone.

is exciting to look at any current issues of alth trade magazines and reports as it s that every month they have new eries and information about the positive that omega-3 has on our bodies, ental outlook and quality of life.

Fiber and Chia

Many of us associate fiber with increased time in the bathroom, but fiber also acts as a speed control in your GI tact or intestine. Just like a speed bump, fiber slows everything down as it travels thorough the digestive tract, slowing the travel time of the food across the ileocecal valve and keep the stomach feeling fuller longer. This makes you feel full longer and increases the appetite suppressing signals. The daily suggested amount of fiber is around 30 grams; please talk with your health care provider as to what you should be taking.

Studies show that by consuming more fiber at breakfast makes you less hungry in the late afternoon or around the time so many of us snack. Consuming additional fiber is quick and easy – just add chia to oatmeal, whole grains or sprinkle on fruits. Those foods are already a great source of fiber just enhanced with chia.

Besides controlling blood sugar levels and decreasing insulin levels, fiber also reduces calorie intake for up to 18 hours a day! One study showed that taking as little as 1 gram of fiber an hour before meals resulted in a weight loss of almost 6 pounds in 8 weeks.

The fiber products that you mix with water that are available at the drug stores are an excellent source of dietary fiber but have very little other vitamins and minerals. Chia costs less, contents fiber and is an excellent source of many needed vitamins and minerals. Why spend money on an empty food source?

Since chia is a food product and is a natural, safe food so you cannot "over doses" on it. If you eat too much you will simply spend a little more time in the bathroom and then can adjust the amount of chia you take.

Do you remember the old saying of "is one prune not enough, is six too many?" That saying can also relate to chia seeds! The suggested daily intake of chia seeds is four teaspoons; since chia is a food product and is a natural, safe food so you can't "over dose" on it. You will simply spend a little more time in the bathroom and know that your body needs a little less or possibly a little more.

Chia also is filled extra vitamins and minerals unlike most other fiber products. Chia is a healthier choice.

Chia is easy to use, just add the desired amount to your breakfast smoothie, cereal, sprinkle it on toast, or maybe just stir it into your orange juice or other juices. Concerned about the gelling properties? Simply heat a small pan over low heat and lightly toast the chia seeds. That will stop the gelling and can be stored for weeks in an airtight container.

Chia is safe, easy to use and an effective source of fiber to maintain your health, stabilize blood sugar and in weight control.

Vitamins and Minerals in Chia

Chia is packed full of vitamins and minerals that are essential to our health and well being. Using chia as part of a balanced and healthy diet will not only increase the fiber and omega-3 but will add all of the following to your body and mental health.

Boron

Boron is considered an ultra trace element required for maintaining the integrity of cell walls. Nearly all plants have some levels of boron depending on the soil conditions and all food from plants contains some levels of boron. Sadly in the world today many regions are becoming boron depleted meaning that many foods are lacking in the necessary boron levels to promote health and to promote good skin and hair quality.

 The US National Institute of Health states that the total daily boron intake in a normal human diet should range between 2.1 and 4.3 mg daily.   Chia contains approximately 1.4 mg boron per 100 grams of chia.

Past research showed that boron is essential for post-menopausal women.   Studies have also suggested that women who needed estrogen replacement therapy could use boron supplement instead.   The newer studies have not proved this theory and boron supplements or boron rich foods could not be used as an estrogen replacement therapy.

Limited studies have shown some improvement of calcium retention in bones with an increase of boron in the diet – more studies need to be conducted before a conclusion can be made.

Boron studies have also showed improvement in copper retention again more studies are necessary before a conclusion can be published.

Copper

Copper is an essential element in all plants and animals. Biologically, copper is used for electron transport within the bloodstream. The recommended daily value is .9mg per day while professional research recommends 3.0 mg per day. Copper deficiency can produce anemia-like symptoms while too much copper can produce Wilson's disease symptoms.

 Foods rich in copper should not be eaten with any diary or egg products as they block copper absorption.

Chia has only trace amounts of copper .2mg per 100 grams of chia.

Sodium

Chia does not contain any sodium. Since most diets contain too much sodium and many Doctors suggesting that we should watch our daily sodium intake this adds to chia being a super power food.

Iron

Iron is essential to most plants and animals and is found mainly in the blood. Iron is part of the many enzymes and proteins that promote and maintain good health by oxygen movement and cell growth. A deficiency of iron results in fatigue and decreased immunity function. 100 grams of chia contains 16.4 mg of iron making chia an excellent source of iron.

According to the Dept. of Agriculture chia is considered an iron-rich food source containing more iron per 100 grams of the edible portion of spinach, lentils, and beef liver.

Zinc

Chia is an excellent source of zinc, a mineral that is essential to maintaining the immune system, digestion, reproduction, diabetes control as well as promoting the health of the prostate, pancreas and salivary gland. Zinc acts as an antioxidant, is a component of many enzyme systems that regulate cell growth, DNA, energy metabolism, hormone levels and growth factor essentials.

Zinc is one of the more important minerals that are essential for protein synthesis which helps regulate the cells in the immune system. By enhancing the immune system, zinc appears to also protect against fungal infections and some infectious diseases such as pneumonia.

Zinc's antioxidant properties help protect cells in the body from free radicals damage. Zinc is also important in protecting the prostate from damage that can lead to inflammation and possible early damage leading to cancer. Along with the metabolism of proteins, lipids, carbohydrates, zinc also is important in the metabolism of vitamin A, cellular immunity, collagen, maintaining taste, maintaining the reproductive organs of both men and woman and to maintaining the proper levels of vitamin E in the body. Studies show that zinc also is part of the regulation of stress levels, the appetite, taste and smell. This mineral is equally important during pregnancy for normal fetus development and for the expectant mother for her health and for development in childhood and early teens.

Chia is high in zinc with 3.7 mg per 100 grams of chia plus suggested protein that studies have shown should be taken with zinc for better absorption. Since chia is also high in protein this is a super food source for the combination.

Manganese

Manganese is found in many food sources so it is rare to see a deviancy in humans. In the body, manganese is found in the bones, liver, pancreas and kidneys and is active in a number of metabolic processes. It helps produce energy from foods, helps the thyroid function and bone formation, and is involved with healing injuries to the muscles.

Diets that are high in animal protein can depleted the body of many minerals including manganese leading to inflammatory diseases and conditions.

Manganese acts as an antioxidant coenzyme that aids in preventing inflammation and other free radicals damage. Ongoing research has determined manganese can improve cognitive skills, reduce irritability and stress; it may also reduce fatigue and weakness in some people. Additional research has shown that manganese can benefit individuals with epilepsy and arthritis.

Chia is an excellent source of manganese with levels of 2.3 mg per 100 grams of chia.

Molybdenum

Molybdenum is a trace element/mineral occurring naturally in spinach and other dark green leafy vegetables, cauliflower, whole grains and legumes. Chia contains .2 mg per 100 grams of chia.

Research shows that only low amounts of molybdenum are needed to help maintain and regulate the ph balance in the body, to increasing nitrogen metabolism and enhance the ability to burn fat.

Molybdenum is necessary in the metabolism of iron and in the working of carrying oxygen to the body's cells and tissues. It also helps eliminate toxic nitrogen waste turning it into uric acid which is then converted and can be flushed from the body.

This trace mineral is found in the kidneys, bones and liver, promotes teeth strength and bone growth. A deficiency may cause impotence. A diet high in processed and refined foods or high in sulfur may decrease molybdenum in the body.

Only a small amount of molybdenum is needed per day, most people do not need to increase their intake.

Niacin called Vitamin B3

Chia is higher in niacin/vitamin B3 than corn, soybeans, rice and safflower. Niacin or vitamin B3 aids the metabolism of food into energy and is found in many grains, dairy, and meats. Niacin also works to decrease the level of cholesterol and fat in the bloodstream. Niacin works to improve the skin, helps to relieve stress and to improve digestion and increase metabolism.

Chia contains 6.13mg of niacin per 100 grams.

Thiamin

Thiamin or vitamin B1 is necessary in energy production and carbohydrate and fatty acid metabolism. Thiamin is responsible for normal development and growth, healthy skin and hair, the immune system to function properly and blood production. One of the major functions of thiamin/vitamin B1 is to maintain the nervous system. People that have celiac disease, chronic diarrhea, colitis, or deficiencies in protein have reduced thiamin absorption. While everyone needs thiamin or B1 daily these people may find they need extra (please talk with your physician).

Chia contains small amounts of thiamin at .18 grams per 100 grams of chia which is similar to rice and corn but lower than soybeans and safflower.

Riboflavin

Riboflavin or vitamin B2 is necessary for the metabolic system and for normal cell growth and function and energy production. Limited research suggests that B2 might be needed in anemia and sickle cell anemia with more research being conducted. It has also been found that people with eating disorders can be deficient in riboflavin.

Chia contents similar percentages of riboflavin as rice and corn with .04 grams per 100 grams of chia.

Vitamin A

Vitamin A is vital for vision, bone growth, cell production, muscles, tissues, lungs and to prevent and fight off infections and viruses. Vitamin A is needed to protect the linings in the eye, lungs, intestines, urinary system and lungs. New research is underway that suggests that Vitamin A is as important as vitamin D to fight off bacterial infections, for the central nervous system and even in weight loss. These studies are still ongoing.

Chia compares with most other grains as to the vitamin A content with 44 IU's per 100 grams of chia.

Calcium

According to a US Department of Agricultural report published in 2002, chia seed contains 6 times more calcium than milk. Calcium is used by the body in both bones and teeth health but is also need for muscle, blood vessels, the secretion of hormones and enzymes and for the nervous system. Calcium is vital for children, aging adults and people with immune diseases.

Chia can provide an excellent source of calcium for all individuals no matter the diet restrictions. Chia is vegan, Kosher, non-dairy and a healthy alternative for calcium and other nutrients. Chia is easy to incorporate into most diets.

There are 714 mg of calcium per 100 grams of chia.

Potassium

Potassium is a heart healthy mineral but is also vital for bones, kidney function, cardiac, skeletal and muscles. Older people should be more concerned with potassium as many of the medicines interfere with potassium absorption as well as their diets are usually lower in potassium. Low levels of potassium can account for high blood pressure, stroke, inflammatory bowel disease (such as Cohn's) and asthma. Potassium levels can also decrease when using certain diuretics and asthma medicines, corticosteroids, antacids, insulin, and laxatives. Please talk to your Doctor if you are concerned about your potassium levels.

Chia contains 700 mg of potassium per 100 grams chia and at least 4 to 6 times the potassium found in milk.

Magnesium

Magnesium is essential for great health and bone structure and is necessary for over 300 biochemical functions in the body. Magnesium helps to regulate blood sugar, normal blood pressure, the immune system, muscle functions, energy metabolism, to prevent cardiovascular diseases, nerve functions. Dietary magnesium is absorbed in the small intestines and as such daily fiber is important to "hold" the magnesium longer for absorption.

Chia seeds are an excellent source of magnesium, containing more magnesium than broccoli.

Phosphorus

Phosphorus is used by the body to replace cells to produce energy, in maintenance of the DNA and RNA structures, to repair bone damage, to strengthen bones and teeth, and to process fats. This mineral is needed to balance other minerals in the body and to metabolize fats and sugars in the body.

Chia seeds are rich in phosphorus with 1,067 mg per 100 grams of chia.

In summary chia is truly a super power food for modern times. Chia is packed full of health benefits, is gluten free, heart healthy and easy to incorporate into your daily diet.

Precautions / Side Effects of Omega-3

Chia seed or oil has no known side effects or allergic reactions. Since chia is so high in omega-3 there are precautions of taken ANY addition food or supplement that contains omega-3. As with all supplements, please check with your health care provider.

People that bruise easily, having any type of bleeding disorder or taking blood thinning medicines that include Coumadin, warfain, or Plavix should limit their omega-3 daily intake to around 3 grams or less per day of omega-3. This is equivalent to three servings of fish per day. For most of us, this should not be a problem but again please check with you health care provider.

Current research reports that omega-3 can reduce the risk of macular degeneration (an eye condition) but that the omega-3 should be fish oil, chia seed or chia oil as it converts into the needed essential fatty acids in the body.

Similar studies have found prostate cancer patients respond in a similar way to omega-3 with the source being fish oil, chia seed or chia oil.

If you are taking any blood sugar lowering medications such as glipizide, Glucotrol or Glucotrol XL, glyburide or insulin some types of omega-3 supplements may increase the need for the medications. Current research shows that chia seed or oil doesn't seem to have the same effect as other forms of omega-3. Check with your health care provider if you start using chia.

Transplant patients that are taking forms of cyclosporine medicine and omega-3 from a safe, pure source may reduce the toxic side effects of the medicine.

Omega-3 added to drug therapy for psoriasis appears to improve the condition.

By increasing the omega-3 fatty acids and decreasing the omega-6 plus following dietary guidelines statins or cholesterol lowing medications may work more effectively.

Studies are showing that increasing the omega-3 fatty acids while taking anti-inflammatory medicines such as Motrin, Advil, Alleve and prescription medicines seem to lower the risk of ulcers. More studies need to be conducted.

As always if you have a medical condition, please consult with your health care provider before changing your diet. Research is showing that not all sources of omega-3 are the same yet chia is the best one available not just today but for the future.

What Can Chia Do For You?

It Starts Before Birth!

As babies develop in their Mother's womb their brains, nervous system and internal organs are growing and of course Mom is losing some vitamins and minerals in the process. A healthy and balanced diet is critical to both Mother and child.

Research has found that adding omega-3 to the Mother's diet is critical for her health and equally important for the health of the child. Researchers at the Boston College Children's Hospital recently released a study of pregnant women that added omega-3 to their normal diet. Following birth these babies performed much better in vision tests with the results noticeable at two months of age. Babies who's Mothers didn't supplement with omega-3 did not do nearly as well on the vision tests. More research is currently underway with those results to be published in about two to three years.

Since chia seed and oil is a food and easy to digest, it can be included in many infant's diets at a very earlier age and should be part of Mother's diet.

Children 18 or younger

The levels of omega-3 daily intake have not been determined for children. Since fish oil can contain contaminants including mercury is not recommended for developing children. Some infant formulas are now being marketed with omega-3. It is suggested that you check with your infant's health care provider prior to using these types of formulas or other enriched youth foods since no effective guidelines for daily usage has been established. You would also want to verify the source of the omega-3 being used. As your children get older, chia is well tolerated, the taste is great and kids of all ages enjoy drinking the chia gel.

Children need the omega-3 balance to omega-6 for healthy development of the brain and nervous systems. The intake of chia can help with attention deficit hypertension ADHD and some behavior problems.

Many children are prone to constipation; chia is a great form of dietary fiber that will help this problem. Chia is rich in protein, boron, calcium and other vitamins and minerals that developing and growing bodies need to become health and strong adults.

A recent Children's Nutrition Survey shows that a majority of parents are not aware of the benefits that DHA has on children, pre-natal and post-natal care or on the unborn child. These same parents did supplement the children's diet with a multi-vitamin and other nutrients such as vitamin C and calcium.

For babies chia oil is a wonderful replacement for baby oil. The chia oil absorbs quickly without a greasy or oily residue plus the omega-3 and other nutrients will be passed through the skin into the body.

The Active Years

During the late teens, twenties and early thirties, we tend to be active, running, jogging, into sports, late hours, early getting up for work, juggling a job and a family. Who has time for diet concerns?

This is the time we should be laying the ground work for those later years in life. You know the routine – daily exercise, a healthy diet, and lots of water. Most people have a hard time even eating a healthy breakfast much less thinking of a balanced life style.

Chia to the rescue!!

Just add a scoop of chia seed to that cereal, sprinkle it on your toast or add it to your smoothie and you are good to go for the rest of the day.

Remember all those Aztec warriors from the beginning of our story? They used chia seeds for endurance and energy. Chia will provide extra athletic endurance in any of your activities even if that's running after the kids. Think what chia can do in a marathon, basketball court or football. Maybe even a birdie or two in your golf game.

The Later Years

The later years are after 40, the time when our body and minds start to slow up and health problems seem to be around every corner.

Chia can help maintain a healthy body, healthy mind and even healthy eyes. As you have been reading, just a little chia daily, about 4 teaspoons, can change the way your body will age. Chia does not cure any disease, does not make you younger, and does not make you dance a jig better. Yet chia provides extra vitamins, minerals and health benefits that will make you live healthier.

As shown chia can make some medicines work a little better or not have some of the side effects that can make life unpleasant. According to most research omega-3 keeps the mind and nerves system working better longer and your eye sight might stay sharp longer.

Chia might not bring us youth but it might help us maintain good health in our later years.

What Diseases/Disorders does Chia Help?

Before we begin, it should be noted that chia is not a miracle "drug" or a cure. Chia is a nutrient packed food. I was speaking with an older gentleman on a Thursday about chia and the health benefits, he asked a few questions, purchased a small amount of chia maybe one pound and left. The following Monday, he called to ask "why haven't I seen the benefits of chia? Well I guess it is just another hyped product!" and hung up the phone. Sadly he didn't want to hear that chia is a food and as a food you may not see any difference in your outer appearance or you might notice your hair is shinier or your skin is softer and natural products will take at least 30 days before noticeable changes occur.

You might notice you have more energy, more vim as they say or a zip in your step as you walk. Dogs and cats react to a chia intake faster than humans. Why? They are a small body mass! For them it usually takes just a few days for us to notice a difference. But since humans are just a little bigger, it takes several weeks before you will notice much difference.

If you are a healthy adult, you might not notice any difference. That does not mean that the body cells, your brain, the nervous system and all your other body parts are not functioning better.

Acne

Acne is skin condition that generally is blocked pores usually caused when the skin follicles become blocked and inflamed. While we think of acne as a teenage condition, many adults are also affected. Studies have shown that in many causes a low sugar diet can help. The dietary studies have also showed that many acne patients also have low levels of zinc. Since chia contains high amounts of zinc, adding chia to your daily diet might improve your acne.

Alzheimer's Disease

Alzheimer's disease, just saying the name causes fear and sadness to most of us, yet it is the seventh leading cause of death in the United State and over five million Americans are living with the disease (according to the National Alzheimer's Association at www.alz.org).

Alzheimer's disease (AD) is a neurodegenerative disease that destroys the brain cells and resulting in memory loss, problems with thinking and behavior. It is a progressive disease without a known cure. Generally it affect men and women 65 years and older but an early onset form does exits.

According to a Norway study published in the Journal of Neurochemistry, patients that increased their daily intake of omega-3 essential fatty acids had a reduction in the declining rate of mental functions in patients over an eight to 12 month period.

Another study at the UCLA showed that individuals who increased their omega-3 DHA levels reduced the mental plaque buildup by 40.3 percent.

Another study at Radbound University Nijmegen, Netherland found that in high risk patients omega-3 did not protect against Alzheimer's. Yet that same study found that normal individuals did receive cognitive benefits from a high omega-3 daily intake and lowering the omega-6 daily intake.

In summary, omega-3 probably will not protect a person from getting Alzheimer's but it might slow the progression or in many people will help maintain mental clarity longer.

Anxiety

Anxiety is a general condition that affects millions of people, from just the occasional bouts to major problems that require a health care provider and prescription medicines.

Some foods seem to enhance or trigger anxiety and include caffeine, alcohol, sugar and other refined foods, other foods to avoid may be dairy, soy, citrus, peanuts and other nuts, fish, corn, wheat, and other foods that are associated with food allergies.

It is also suggested that the diet include more calcium, magnesium and vitamin B complex to help support the nervous system.

Chia is an excellent source of calcium and magnesium.

Asthma

Clinical studies are reporting that omega-3 fatty acids may decrease the inflammation and improve lung functions while omega-6 fatty acids have the opposite effect. When the omega-6 has decreased to the proper ratio to omega-3 the results were quite impressive. When the omega-6 was increased there was an increase and worsening of the respiratory problems.

Results show decrease the omega-6 and increase the omega-3 and the simplest, easy way is chia.

Attention Deficit / Hyperactivity Disorder (ADHD)

ADHD is one of the most common neurobehavioral disorders in children and the cause of the disease is not known. What is known is that certain foods can make the problem much worst.

It has been found in several clinical studies that adding omega-3 to the diet helps most patients. Because chia is so high in omega-3 and is easy to use, children respond well to the taste and chia is so nutrient rich it is a great choice.

Autism

Autism is an incurable mental disorder with unknown causes. There are a number of on-going studies is to what is best treatment. Many of the newer treatments include nutrient based care and omega-3 is being proven to have many benefits. Children have been shown to improve dramatically using omega-3 from fish oil with newer studies on-going comparing those results with chia. Chia is of course much safer to use than fish oil yet has the same type of omega-3, easier to digest, and easy to use.

Research shows that about 50% of patients with Autism cannot break down gluten and the casein proteins with some of those proteins entering the bloodstream. Gluten and casein free foods seem to decrease the symptoms in those individuals.

Chia is gluten and casein free.

Bi-Polar Disorder

Bi-polar disorder is another neuro-disorder that strikes all ages and both genders. The medicine that is prescribed can cause a loss of appetite and a loss of nutrients within the body leading to other health problems.

Studies have shown that an increase of omega-3 in the diet while decreasing the omega-6 can help the medicine work better and have fewer mood swings. Of course chia is high in omega-3 and all the other good stuff that our bodies need to function. More research is being conducted with chia as the omega-3 source and findings should be published in the next year to two years.

Burns / Rashes and Other Skin Problems

Research is currently being conducted to determine just how omega-3 and proteins help to heal burns, rashes and other skin problems.

The few studies that have been reported show that omega-3 helps to reduce the inflammation of the skin, promoting healing. They have also found a balance of protein in the body is necessary to promote the healing of burns.

We have had a number of reports from individuals with various types of skin problems including cement burns (cement workers), dry skin, unknown rashes that Doctors have not been able to diagnosis, psoriasis and just plain it itches to be helped using chia. Some of the people have used the gel caps, others take the seeds with a meal and others slather on the chia oil straight from the bottle or with a cotton tip swab dabbed onto the area. The reports back from these folk are really amazing and wonderful! They tell us about how they have not felt this good in years. The red spots are gone, the itching is not there, and one young man was no longer embarrassed in the locker room at school because of his psoriasis.

Will it work for you? Maybe, we suggest you try it and then report back to us.

Cancer

Most cancer patients are told to consume less red meat, less diary, eggs, and to increase their intake of vegetables, beans, foods that have antioxidants, etc. Many of the medicines that are being taken cause a loss of appetite. What can be done?

Chia is, of course, high in protein, high in antioxidants, easy to digest and has the needed fiber to move things along.

Chia is easy to mix into other foods or can be stirred into a glass of liquid.

Crohn's Disease and Gluten Intolerance

While Crohn's disease and gluten intolerance are not the same disease, they share many of the symptoms and they both affect the intestine, the tissues of the intestine, diarrhea, and other nasty problems.

Many of the same foods are culprits and are to be taken out of the diet. Most of those foods are high in protein, calcium, vitamins and minerals. Removing them from the diet then causes other problems. To make it worst, the person is told to increase their fiber intake!

Once again super power food chia to the rescue!! Chia, as you know, is high in all the good things yet is gluten free. Plus chia is easily tolerated by all ages.

Diabetes

Much information has been written about chia and diabetes yet few studies have actually been done. Chia probably does help to stabilize the blood sugar simply because the food is keep in the digestive tract longer, it also helps move the nutrients between the cell walls better.

The American Diabetes Association recommends diabetics to eat a low-fat diet that is rich in grains, fruits and vegetables with between 10-20 percent of calories from protein including fish. This will almost help to lower blood pressure and cholesterol as well as controlling blood sugars.

Chia will not lower your blood sugar; it will help you eat a healthy diet low in fats, with protein and calcium. Since chia is low in cholesterol it is a good source of all the vitamins and minerals that constitute a healthy diet. Since chia also has a high fiber content, the foods will move thorough the digestive tract better.

Depression

If a health ratio of omega-3 to omega-6 is not included in a diet or if the omega-3 level is low there appears to be a higher risk of depression. Omega-3 fatty acids are important in the way the nerve cell membranes communicate with each other. In one clinical study, subjects that increased their intake of omega-3 experienced a significant decrease in feelings of depression and hostility.

High Cholesterol

As we know, people that eat a Mediterranean type diet tend to have lower cholesterol levels. People that eat a lot of fish that contain high amounts of omega-3 fatty acids also have high HDL cholesterol (that's the good stuff) and lower triglycerides (that's the bad stuff). The bad news about this is that many of the fish oils are not the highest amounts of omega-3 and may not be pure and natural or even contain cholesterol!

The body treats chia just as it does fish oil so you get all the "good stuff" without any of the "bad stuff". Plus you only have to add a small amount of chia into your daily diet to experience many health benefits.

Several clinical trials have shown that Chia or Salvia Hispanica can help lower triglyceride levels. Salvia Hispanica was shown to lower the levels more than any other source of omega-3. When fish oil was studied it did lower the triglyceride levels by 25 percent but it increased the LDL levels by 22 percent in only the first six weeks of the study.

Chia lowered both the total cholesterol and the LDL cholesterol, and triglycerides with the optimal dosage of 30 grams of seed or oil per day.

Further studies are still on-going.

High Blood Pressure

Seventeen different clinical studies show that diets high in certain types of omega-3 (fish oil was used) can significantly reduce blood pressure in people with untreated high blood pressure.

Since chia seeds and oil contain the same type of omega-3 as fish oil, chia would be a great option.

Macular Degeneration

Macular degeneration is a degenerative and painless disease of the eyes that affects millions of people over the age of 55 and is the leading cause of blindness in that age group.

There is no known cure for macular generation but there are ways to slow the loss of vision. Please consult with your eye care provider.

Once again a healthy diet has been found to help slow the process. Over eighteen different studies have found that a diet rich in antioxidants, zinc, vitamins C and E and omega-3 are especially important to add to the diet.

In one study of over 3,000 people omega-3 from fish oil (remember chia is metabolic similar to fish oil) was added to their diets. The results showed these people were less likely to develop macular degeneration than people that did not increase the omega-3 from fish oil. Addition studies found that lowering the omega-6 intake and increasing the healthy omega-3 intake, the subjects again slowed the progress of the disease or did not have the disease.

This is another reason to include chia seeds and oil into your diet.

Menstrual Pain

A Danish clinical study of about two hundred women showed that those with high omega-3 levels in their diet had the mildest menstrual pain. More research is currently on-going.

Menopause

The Danish clinical study mentioned above also includes women that were earlier menopausal. Again, women with high omega-3 levels had reduced hot flashes, less symptoms, and better sleeping patterns.

Several years ago, there was a report that boron or boron enriched foods could be used as an estrogen replacement therapy, this has been found incorrect. While boron helps the density of bones it is NOT a replacement therapy. Additionally chia does not contain any estrogen or any estrogen producing chemical and is safe to consume with any medical estrogen replacement therapy.

Migraine Headaches

Research is finding that many foods are "trigger points" for migraine headaches and are to be eaten with caution. As always please consult with your health care provider about what is best for your care.

Anytime foods are removed from a diet that means there is a potential of other health problems.

It has been found that many people that suffer from migraine headaches are also low in magnesium levels. Limited studies have shown that adding magnesium to the diet or by taking supplements can lower the number of migraines or can help with the severity of the pain in conjunction with the medicine.

Chia is rich in magnesium! Since magnesium just might stop those headaches why not add chia to your diet?

Osteoarthritis / Rheumatoid Arthritis

Osteoarthritis is the most common form of arthritis, making life miserable for millions of people.

Rheumatoid arthritis is a chronic illness that causes inflammation and swelling of the joints and tissues around the joints. In addition rheumatoid arthritis can cause damage to the organs.

Both rheumatoid arthritis and osteoarthritis studies have shown that similar treatments can improve the quality of live.

While there is no cure, we can do things that can make life more comfortable and enjoyable. Sure we all know about glucosamine and chondroitin with many of us adding those supplements, then there are all the over the counter pain medicines that work for some of us or the prescription drugs that might work also.

But did you know that adding omega-3 to your diet will help those medicines work better! Or that the antioxidants found in chia can ease the inflammation caused by free radicals, the same free radicals that can cause degenerative joints?

The omega-3 found in chia can also decrease the inflammation and reduced the activity of enzymes that break down the cartilage.

Osteoporosis

To many of us just the word Osteoporosis sends fear running up and down our spines. While the disease is thought to be an older person's disease, it can strike at any age. The bones lose density or become brittle increasing the risk of fractures. Please consult your health care provider for details and methods of treatment.

Studies suggest that a diet rich in calcium, magnesium, potassium, fruits and vegetables will help. Additional studies show that diets rich in omega-3 fatty acids can help to maintain or even increase the bone mass.

Since chia contains the highest source of omega-3, a great source for both calcium and magnesium it makes sense to add chia to your diet.

Prostate Cancer

I read an article about prostate cancer recently that stated most men will experience some type of prostate problems in their life. These problems can be a simple inflammation, a virus, or sadly prostate cancer.

Research that is currently being conducted is finding that a healthy diet can slow many of the problems. What I found interesting was the healthy diet was based on East Indian food. This means turmeric, cumin, curry powders, fish, lean red meat, chicken and rice. The same study then added omega-3 from fish oils (once again remember that chia contains the same type of omega-3) and were surprised to learn that omega-3 played a huge part in reducing the occurrence of prostate problems!

Just another reason to add chia to your daily diet!

Weight Loss

We have been asked a number of questions about chia and weight loss.

Very important --- chia does not cause you to lose weight!! It is not a weight loss supplement or diet pill. If you have a medical condition and are very thin, you will not lose weight consuming either the chia seed or oil.

What chia seed does do is make a person feel fuller longer. Since you feel fuller, it decreases the trigger to snack. If your medical condition requires snacks or several light meals, chia seed will not interfere with those yet will add a lot of extra vitamins and minerals.

Chia Seed Oil

Chia seed can be cold pressed, similar to the way olive oil is pressed, producing slightly nutty smelling golden oil. This oil is then either processed into gel caps as an omega-3 supplement or left as a liquid.

Chia oil contains all the good for you vitamins and minerals of the seed, with the only difference is the oil does not contain the seeds fiber. The seeds are then toasted, ground into a powder and used in other products. The chia meal or powder contains some left over nutrients but the levels are fairly low and this product is used mainly for sport drinks, baby foods as part of nutrimental profile not as a standalone good for you product like either the seeds or oil.

The pleasant flavor, nutty smelling oil can be used as in salad dressing mix, drizzled onto food, or as a body care product or part of a body care product.

Any oil that contains high amounts of omega-3 fatty essential acids should not be used as cooking oil, since the fatty essential acids will oxidative.

You can use chia oil instead of olive oil in salad dressing. Use it as a dipping sauce with minced garlic, dipping a piece of crusty bread into the oil. For people that have problems eating solid foods, chia oil can be added to soft foods such as mashed carrots, cereals, or even apple sauce. The possibilities are limited to the foods served.

In the book "Cooking with Chia" there are a number of recipes that incorporate chia oil into everyday recipes.

As stated chia oil is packed full of the same nutrients as the seed and can be used by the teaspoon by mouth if desired. Many vegans prefer using the oil in this manner, or if you have health issues that may stop you from taking the gel caps or the seeds.

Anything that is used on the skin will be absorbed by the skin into the blood system and cells of the body. This ability of the skin is why you need to use all natural body care products.

When chia oil is used directly on the skin it is non-greasy or oily feeling (men like this), it absorbs rapidly into the skin with no sticky residue. As chia oil is absorbed so are all the omega-3, vitamins, minerals, protein, etc. Those elements are like food to the skin cells. The cells will respond with better health, less dry skin and better cellular structure. This is also a great way to increase the nutrients to the rest of the body.

Rashes, burns and some skin problems such as fungi can also be helped with the use of chia oil. As always please consult with your health care provider before using.

Some people like to use chia oil as part of their hair shampooing routine, as it hydrates the scalp and hair. A small amount used by its self or mixed with your favorite shampoo will work very well.

Chia oil can also be used as an ingredient in most body care products or massage oil. Use either your recipe to produce the care products using chia oil instead of say sweet almond oil. Or you can mix chia oil into your favorite cream or lotion, and then apply to your skin.

As you can see – chia oil is not just for food or a dietary supplement.

Amaranth and Chia

Almost everything that has been written about chia states "chia, amaranth and maize were staple foods of the Aztecs", it was decided that a section about amaranth should be added to these book.

Amaranth and chia were staple crops of the ancient Aztecs and both were grown at least 8,000 years ago. Amaranth was considered as valuable as chia and was presented to the Aztec leaders for payment of taxes. Both crops were used in religious ceremonies, and just as chia, were suppressed by the Spanish invaders. About twenty years ago the National Academy of Sciences recommended Amaranth as one of the twenty foods that could be reintroduced into the modern diet.

Amaranth is high in dietary fiber, iron, calcium, lysine, methhionine, cysteine and protein. It is very low in sodium and contains no saturated fat. Amaranth is gluten free, vegetarian and heart healthy.

Amaranth leaves are also eaten and are similar to spinach and can be used to replace spinach in recipes or salads.

The name amaranth comes from the Greek word amarantus which means "never fading flower". The plant is an annual herb and not a true grain such as wheat or barley, the plant is a relative of the common pigweed also know as lamb's quarters and cockscomb. There are over sixty species of amaranth and all can be used for food including the leaves and the seeds.

Amaranth plants resist heat, drought, has no disease problems, is easy to grow and is found in many parts of the world. The seeds can be used as a cereal either alone or with other seeds/grains, popped similar to popcorn, used in soups, stir fry, or in granola type products. The seeds can be ground into delicious flour for all type of baked goods, tortillas, pancakes, flatbreads or pastas. The seeds can be easily sprouted and used in sandwiches.

While we think of Mexico as the country that mainly uses amaranth; various cultures are using the plant is some unique culinary dishes. In Peru the seed is fermented to make "chichi" or what is known as a type of beer. The leaves are cooked as a vegetable in Peru and eaten either boiled or fried. In India the "rajerra" or Kings' grain as amaranth is called is popped and used in a number of candies. "Sattoo" is gruel type cereal made with grounded seeds in Nepal. In other places, including Ecuador, the flowers are used as a type of food coloring or as a medicine to purify the blood.

Amaranth seeds can be found in most health food stores or the natural product section in the grocery store. Amaranth is slowly gaining popularity as it is high in protein, has vitamin E, vitamin C vitamin A, high in iron, two times more calcium than milk, high levels of potassium and phosphorus, and contains no gluten.

Chia and amaranth have been used together for centuries. Chia maintains the energy levels for long periods of time while amaranth provides a boost of energy when consumed. Both have been mixed together and eaten as cereal type foods or ground together to produce flours for breads.

The two grain-like seeds made for some tasty additions to a modern diet. Check out just a few recipes in the following section.

Basic Amaranth Recipe

Makes 1 ½ cups

1 ½ cup water

½ cup amaranth

In a small saucepan, over medium heat combine the

Cover and boil for about 20 minutes until all the water is absorbed. Be careful to not overcook as amaranth will become a little mushy.

The amaranth is now ready to enjoy. Eat as you would rice, in a salad, with a little milk and/or sugar for a breakfast treat or desert. Add a couple of teaspoons of chia for crunch and added nutrients.

Popped Amaranth

This can be dangerous! So get out the skillet lid, protective glasses and even the oven mitts!

¼ cup amaranth seeds (or the amount called from in your recipe)

1 skillet do not use non-stick since this is a dry skillet over very high heat.

Over high heat, place the skillet on the element or burner and heat until it is very hot. Water will dance on the surface hot. Add in the amaranth and watch it pop all over the place. The seeds will act like popcorn does in a skillet. Stir constantly until all the seeds are popped and a golden brown. Be careful not to burn the seeds. Pour the popped amaranth into a bowl until ready to use.

The amaranth can be eaten just as it is, or you can add fruit, or milk, or you can be creative.

Chia Gel

One of the most popular ways to use chia is to create chia gel.

Place one part chia to nine part of a liquid normally water but it can be any non-citrus liquid into a container, stir and let set for about 10 minutes. An example of the "parts" is 1 ounce of chia seed to 8 ounces of liquid. After 10 to 15 minutes, stir again to break up any clumps. The chia gel is ready to use. Store in a covered container for up to two weeks in the refrigerator.

Toasted Chia Seeds

Chia seeds do not need to be ground or cracked before using. Toasting chia seeds will stop them from forming the above gel and can add a crunch to many dishes or salads.

To toast, place a small non-stick skillet over high heat. When the skillet is nice and hot, add the amount of chia seeds you would like to toast and stir to prevent the seeds from burning until you can smell them – about 4 minutes. Cool and store in an air tight container using as desired.

Amaranth & Chia Breakfast Cereal

This recipe is filled with goodness plus the fiber of the chia and prunes.

3 tablespoons chia seed

1 cup water

3 cups amaranth seed

¼ cup chopped prunes

1/8 cup chopped walnuts

1 teaspoon cinnamon

Serve with milk of your choice

In a small bowl, stir the chia seeds into the water and set aside for about 15 minutes until gelled.

In a large saucepan over medium heat cook the 3 cups of amaranth in 6 cups of water. Cook about 20 minutes or until the water is mostly absorbed. Add all the other ingredients, stir lightly until mixed. Place into serving bowls. Add milk and sugar if desired.

Chia and Amaranth Pancakes

1 egg beaten

¼ cup milk of your choice or water

1 teaspoon oil

½ cup amaranth flour

2 tablespoons chia seed

Pinch of salt

1 teaspoon baking power

Makes 10 pancakes 3 inches in diameter

In a medium mixing bowl, add the beaten egg and mix in the water or milk, the oil and mix well. Add the remaining ingredients one by one in any order but mix each addition well before adding the next.

Heat a pan or griddle over medium heat until hot. Pour the batter onto to hot griddle into small pancakes, flipping after bubbles form.

Usually about two minutes per side. Serve hot with butter, syrup, honey.

Amaranth & Chia Pudding

Makes 8 – ½ cup servings

1 cup amaranth seeds

¼ cup chia seed

3 cups of milk of your choice

1 cup coconut unsweetened

 1 teaspoon vanilla

½ cup sweeter – honey, sugar or other choice

Pinch of salt

Heat the oven to 350 degrees

In a large saucepan over medium heat, heat the milk until scalded. Add all the other ingredients to the milk and stir well.

Pour the milk mixture into a greased or sprayed casserole dish. Place the casserole into the oven. Bake for 1 hour.

Serve hot or cold. Can be served with berries, whipped cream or in any similar fashion to rice pudding.

Quick White Bean Soup

Makes 4 cups

½ cup amaranth seed

¼ cup chia seed

2 cloves of garlic minced

2 leeks, white parts only, cleaned and sliced

3 cups chicken stock, vegetable stock or water

2 tablespoons olive oil or other cooking oil

1 cup or 1 can chopped tomatoes

1 can (15 ounce) white kidney beans or cannellini beans drained – divide into two containers

2 teaspoons each dried oregano and dried basil or Italian seasoning

Salt and black pepper to taste.

In a medium saucepan, sauté the leeks in the olive oil until they are golden brown and soft, app. 10 minutes. Add the garlic until soft but not brown. Add the amaranth, chicken stock and tomatoes and bring to a boil. Reduce the heat to a simmer, cover and cook for 20 minutes or until the amaranth has absorbed the liquid.

Place half of the beans into a blender, blend until smooth. Add the cooked amaranth mixture and puree. Pour the puree back into the saucepan, stir in the remaining beans and chia, heat until warm. Season with the dried herbs, salt and pepper.

Serve hot.

Chia & Amaranth Salad Dressing

½ cup popped amaranth

½ cup toasted chia seeds

1 cup olive or vegetable oil

1 tablespoon soy salt (low sodium if available)

3 garlic cloves minced or pressed

Mix all the ingredients in a container. Cover and refrigerate overnight for the flavors to blend.

Use as desired on a vegetable or pasta salad or even as a sauce for chicken or fish.

Chicken in Chia & Amaranth Sauce

Serves 4

We have found the sauce is so much better if you make it the day before, then the day of serving brown the chicken, onions and add the sauce and continue as stated.

3 tablespoons cooking oil

4 boneless, skinless chicken breasts (we like to pound the chicken flat prior to cooking as this evens out the thickness so it cooks better – just use a meat mallet, put a chicken piece into a plastic bag and lightly pound until the thickness desired)

2 onions peeled and sliced thin

4 cloves finely chopped garlic

1 can chopped tomatoes with juice

½ chipotle chili with a small amount of the adobo sauce – this can be omitted or increased per taste

1 can chicken broth

¼ cup amaranth seeds

¼ cup chia seeds

Heat a large skillet over high heat. When hot add the amaranth seeds and pop like popcorn, until the seeds are all white and fluffy. Pour the seeds into a blender. In the same skillet toast the chia seeds until you can smell the toasty aroma, pour the chia seeds into the blender.

Using the same skillet, lower the heat to medium high, add the cooking oil and brown the chicken on both sides. When finished, move the chicken to a plate for later.

If needed, add more cooking oil and sauté the onions and garlic until the onions are soft but not completely cooked.

As the onions are cooking, put the tomato, chicken stock and chipotles (if using) into the blender with the amaranth and chia seeds. Blend until a thick puree.

Add the puree mixture to the cooking onions and stir until combined.

At this point, the sauce can be cooled and refrigerated for up to 3 days.

Reheat the sauce if needed.

Add the browned chicken to the sauce and cook for about 20 minutes until the chicken is no longer pink inside.

Remove the chicken to a serving platter. Put the sauce into a serving bowl. Serve with rice using the sauce over the chicken and rice.

Amaranth Tortillas

This recipe does not contain any chia seeds but it is included to show how the ancient foods are still popular today. This might have been a staple food in most Aztec homes.

Make about 6 tortillas

1 ¼ cups amaranth flour

½ cup water

In a small bowl mix the amaranth flour and water until the dough is soft and molds easily into shapes. Add a bit more flour or water to get the proper consistency.

Make size golf ball size balls of dough. Roll them in a little amaranth flour, knead each ball several times as you either pat it or roll it into a flat circle about 1/8 inch thick, 5 inches in diameter.

Heat a non-stick frying pan or griddle. No oil is required.

Cook one tortilla at a time about 2 minutes per side. Cool on a wire rack.

Serve hot or store in the refrigerator for up to 2 weeks. Reheat before using.

Chia BBQ Sauce

We love to smoke foods! You name it and we've probably smoked it from cheese to fruit to fish. And what is smoked or grilled food without the BBQ sauce? The down side to this is that most sauces are high calorie with lots of sugars so what can you do to maintain a healthy diet? Chia to the rescue!

Make chia gel and mix with the BBQ sauce. Just make equal portions of chia gel to the BBQ sauce, stir together and serve. You can use any BBQ sauce you like from home made to store brought.

Chia Compound Butter

Compound butter is just softened butter with herbs, or garlic, or honey or you can use your imagination to create your families favorite.

We like garlic bread with many pasta dishes so have compound butters stored in the freezer.

Sadly butter is fat, even the low-cal spreads are still not really healthy but taste so good.

Again chia to the rescue!!

To whip up some tasty healthy spread, just soften the butter or spread at room temperature, using either a mixing spoon, blender, or electric mixer mix the butter, herb or garlic or honey into the butter. Then add an equal portion of the chia gel, mix well. Place the butter mixture onto a piece of plastic wrap or wax paper and form into a log. Roll the paper or wrap tightly and twist the ends tight to seal in the goodness. Store in the freezer until ready to use. Then unroll, slice off what you need, re-roll the rest, popping it back into the freezer. Soften the remainder at room temperature.

Tomato Jam

Tomato jam is wonderful on fish, chicken and even pasta. It is easy to make and you can prepared it all year using either fresh or canned tomatoes.

Seed 4 large meaty tomatoes or use 2 cans of tomatoes drained.

¼ cup onion finely chopped

2 cloves of garlic finely chopped

1 cup chia gel

Juice of 1 lemon

Salt and pepper to taste.

In a nonreactive medium saucepan, add the tomatoes, garlic and onion. Simmer for 20 minutes or until the mixture is reduced to 1 cup. Remove from heat; stir in the chia gel, the lemon juice, salt and pepper. Serve hot or cold. Store in the refrigerator for up to 4 days.

Greek Cucumber Yogurt Sauce

While yogurt is a healthy choice we can make it even healthier with chia gel.

½ cup yogurt

¼ cup chia gel

½ cup peeled grated English or seedless cucumber

Drain the grated cucumber in a small bowl by pressing the cucumber with the back of a wooden spoon, and pouring off the liquid. Mix in the yogurt and chia gel. Store in the refrigerator until ready to serve. Will keep about 3 days. Great with lamb, beef skewers, hamburgers, chicken.

Summer Strawberry Salad

Adapted from Daily Diabetes Care

Summer 2008

1 cup Greek Style yogurt

½ cup chia gel

1 tablespoon orange marmalade

2 pints fresh strawberries, hulled and halved

Pinch of ground nutmeg

In a large bowl, combine the yogurt, chia gel, marmalade and nutmeg. Chill for at least two hours in the refrigerator so the flavors can combine.

To serve, place the strawberries into 6 serving bowls and top with the yogurt mixture.

Quick Yogurt Snack

Mix chia seeds with yogurt and fruit. Easy, fast and a great pick-me-up of energy, protein snack or light lunch.

Smart Summertime Eating

Most of us think that summertime eating is filled with healthy, fresh foods and it can be. Then there are the lemonades, the hamburgers with all the fixin's, the ice cream and we cannot forget the street fairs and country fairs.

To "lighten" the wonderful fresh salads, add chia gel to the salad dressings for half the fat and calories yet with all the taste and a boost in the nutrients.

Add chia gel to the mayo again to half the fat and calories and to sneak in that calcium and fiber.

Add a tablespoon of chia seeds to that lemonade, it won't cut the calories but it will add energy and nutrients on a hot day. Remember those Aztec warriors running thorough the jungles and mountains. Think how much more energy you will have on the golf

Peanut Butter Spread

We like peanut butter but not the fat and calories. What to do?

Make chia gel as per directions. Then mix ½ cup chia gel and ½ cup peanut butter to make 1 cup of healthier peanut butter spread. The spread will have ½ of both calories and fat. This is a great way to get kids to eat a healthier snack.

Fruit Water

4 ounces water

4 ounces of your favorite fruit juice

2 teaspoons of chia seed

Pour the water and fruit juice into a glass, stir in chia and drink. A refreshing change of pace plus a boost of energy from the chia.

Chia Fruit Salad

1 package of mixed salad greens or your choice of greens

1 mango peeled, seeded and diced

1 pound cooked shrimp peeled

8 ounces diced pineapple

8 ounces diced melon of your choice such as watermelon, honeydew or cantaloupe

4 teaspoons of chia

4 tablespoons of Greek style yogurt

4 tablespoons of Dijon style mustard

1 tablespoon honey

4 tablespoons of prepared or homemade vinaigrette dressing

Combine the vinaigrette, mustard, honey and yogurt in a large bowl. Whisk until thorough mixed. Add the rest of the ingredients except the salad greens and toss lightly until all the fruit and shrimp is coated. Refrigerate at least 1 hour to 4 hours. Divide the salad greens onto 4 plates. Divide the fruit and shrimp mixture on top of the greens and serve.

For additional recipes see "Cooking with Chia" available at amazon.com, Borders, Barnes and Noble, and other fine bookstores. Also available at www.chiaforhealth.com

Supporting Research

Office of Dietary Supplements
National Institutes of Health
Bethesda, Maryland 20892 USA

University of Maryland Medical School

22 South Green St

Baltimore MD 21201

Al-Harbi MM, Islam MW, Al-Shabanah OA, Al-Gharably NM. Effect of acute administration of fish oil (omega-3 marine triglyceride) on gastric ulceration and secretion induced by various ulcerogenic and necrotizing agents in rats. *Fed Chem Toxic* . 1995;33(7):555-558.

Albert CM, Hennekens CH, O'Donnell CJ, et al. Fish consumption and risk of sudden cardiac death. *JAMA* . 1998;279(1):23-28.

Ando H, Ryu A, Hashimoto A, Oka M, Ichihashi M. Linoleic acid and alpha-linolenic acid lightens ultraviolet-induced hyperpigmentation of the skin. *Arch Dermatol Res* . 1998;290(7):375-381.

Andreassen AK, Hartmann A, Offstad J, Geiran O, Kvernebo K, Simonsen S. Hypertension prophylaxis with omega-3 fatty acids in heart transplant recipients. *J Am Coll Cardiol.* 1997;29:1324-1331.

Angerer P, von Schacky C. n-3 polyunsaturated fatty acids and the cardiovascular system. *Curr Opin Lipidol* . 2000;11(1):57-63.

Anti M, Armelau F, Marra G, et al. Effects of different doses of fish oil on rectal cell proliferation in patients with sporadic colonic adenomas. *Gastroenterology* . 1994;107(6):1892-1894.

Appel LJ. Nonpharmacologic therapies that reduce blood pressure: a fresh perspective. *Clin Cardiol* . 1999;22(Suppl. III):III1-III5.

Arnold LE, Kleykamp D, Votolato N, Gibson RA, Horrocks L. Potential link between dietary intake of fatty acid and behavior: pilot exploration of serum lipids in attention-deficit hyperactivity disorder. *J Child Adolesc Psychopharmacol* . 1994;4(3):171-182.

Aronson WJ, Glaspy JA, Reddy ST, Reese D, Heber D, Bagga D. Modulation of omega-3/omega-6 polyunsaturated ratios with dietary fish oils in men with prostate cancer. *Urology* . 2001;58(2):283-288.

Badalamenti S, Salerno F, Lorenzano E, et al. Renal Effects of Dietary Supplementation With Fish Oil in Cyclosporine-Treated Liver Transplant Patients. *Hepatol* . 1995;2(6):1695-1701.

Baumgaertel A. Alternative and controversial treatments for attention-deficit/hyperactivity disorder. *Pediatr Clin of North Am* . 1999;46(5):977-992.

Belluzzi A, Boschi S, Brignola C, Munarini A, Cariani C, Miglio F. Polyunsaturated fatty acids and inflammatory bowel disease. *Am J Clin Nutr* . 2000;71(suppl):339S-342S.

Belluzzi A, Brignolia C, Campieri M, Pera A, Boschi S, Miglioli M. Effect of an enteric-coated fish-oil preparation on relapses in Crohn's disease. *New Engl J Med.* 1996;334(24):1558-1560.

Boelsma E, Hendriks HF. Roza L. Nutritional skin care: health effects of micronutrients and fatty acids. *Am J Clin Nutr* . 2001;73(5):853-864.

Bonaa KH, Bjerve KS, Nordoy A. Docosahexaenoic and eicosapentaenoic acids in plasma phospholipids are divergently associated with high density lipoprotein in humans. *Arterioscler Thromb* . 1992;12(6):675-681.

Broadhurst CL, Cunnane SC, Crawford MA. Rift Valley lake fish and shellfish provided brain-specific nutrition for early Homo. *Br J Nutr* . 1998;79(1):3-21.

Brown DJ, Dattner AM. Phytotherapeutic approaches to common dermatologic conditions. *Arch Dermtol* . 1998;134:1401-1404.

Bruinsma KA, Taren DL. Dieting, essential fatty acid intake, and depression. *Nutrition Rev.* 2000;58(4):98-108.

Burgess J, Stevens L, Zhang W, Peck L. Long-chain polyunsaturated fatty acids in children with attention-deficit hyperactivity disorder. *Am J Clin Nutr* . 2000; 71(suppl):327S-330S.

Calder PC. n-3 polyunsaturated fatty acids, inflammation and immunity: pouring oil on troubled waters or another fishy tale? *Nut Res* . 2001;21:309-341.

Caron MF, White CM. Evaluation of the antihyperlipidemic properties of dietary supplements. *Pharmacotherapy* . 2001;21(4):481-487.

Cellini M, Caramazzu N, Mangiafico P, Possati GL, Caramazza R. Fatty acid use in glaucomatous optic neuropathy treatment. *Acta Ophthalmol Scand Suppl* . 1998;227:41-42.

Cho E, Hung S, Willet WC, Spiegelman D, Rimm EB, Seddon JM, et al. Prospective study of dietary fat and the risk of age-related macular degeneration. *Am J Clin Nutr* . 2001;73(2):209-218.

Christensen JH, Skou HA, Fog L, Hansen V, Vesterlund T, Dyerberg J, Toft E, Schmidt EB. Marine n-3 fatty acids, wine intake, and heart rate variability in patients referred for coronary angiography. *Circulation* . 2001;103:623-625.

Clark WF, Kortas C, Heidenheim AP, Garland J, Spanner E, Parbtani A. Flaxseed in lupus nephritis: a two–year nonplacebo-controlled crossover study. *J Am Coll Nutr* . 2001;20(2 Suppl):143-148.

Connolly JM, Gilhooly EM, Rose DP. Effects of reduced dietary linoleic acid intake, alone or combined with an algal source of docosahexaenoic acid, on MDA-MD-231 breast cancer cell growth and apoptosis in nude mice. *Nutrition Can* . 1999;35(1):44-49.

Connor SL, Connor WE. Are fish oils beneficial in the prevention and treatment of coronary artery disease? *Am J Clin Nutr.* 1997;66(suppl):1020S-1031S.

Curtis CL, Hughes CE, Flannery CR, Little CB, Harwood JL, Caterson B. N-3 fatty acids specifically modulate catabolic factors involved in articular cartilage degradation. *J Biol Chem* . 2000;275(2):721-724.

Danao-Camara TC, Shintani TT. The dietary treatment of inflammatory arthritis: case reports and review of the literature. *Hawaii Med J* . 1999;58(5):126-131.

Danno K, Sugie N. Combination therapy with low-dose etretinate and eicosapentaenoic acid for psoriasis vulgaris. *J Dermatol* . 1998;25:703-705.

Davidson MH, Maki KC, Kalkowski J, Schaefer EJ, Torri SA, Drennan KB. Effects of docosahexeaenoic acid on serum lipoproteins in patients with combined hyperlipidemia. A randomized, double-blind, placebo-controlled trial. *J Am Coll Nutr* . 1997;16:3:236-243.

de Deckere EAM. Possible beneficial effect of fish and fish n-3 polyunsaturated fatty acids in breast and colorectal cancer. *Eur J Cancer Prev* . 1999;8:213-221.

deDeckere EAM, Korver O, Verschuren PM, Katan MB. Health aspects of fish and n-3 polyunsaturated fatty acids from plant and marine origin. *Eur J Clin Nutr* . 1998;52(10):749-753.

de Logeril M, Salen P, Martin JL, Monjaud I, Delaye J, Mamelle N. Mediterranean diet, traditional risk factors, and the rate of cardiovascular complications after myocardial infarction: final report of the Lyon Diet Heart Study. *Circulation* . 1999;99(6):779-785.

De-Souza DA, Greene LJ. Pharmacological nutrition after burn injury. *J Nutr.* 1998;128:797-803.

Deutch B. Menstrual pain in Danish women correlated with low n-3 polyunsaturated fatty acid intake. *Eur J Clin Nutr* . 1995;49(7):508-516.

Dewailly E, Blanchet C, Lemieux S, et al. n-3 fatty acids and cardiovascular disease risk factors among the Inuit of Nunavik. *Am J Clin Nutr* . 2001;74(4):464-473.

Dichi I, Frenhane P, Dichi JB, Correa CR, Angeleli AY, Bicudo MH, et al. Comparison of omega-3 fatty acids and sulfasalazine in ulcerative colitis. *Nutrition* . 2000;16:87-90.

Edwards R, Peet M, Shay J, Horrobin D. Omega-3 polyunsaturated fatty acid levels in the diet and in red blood cell membranes of depressed patients. *J Affect Disord* . 1998;48(2-3):149-155.

Fatty fish consumption and ischemic heart disease mortality in older adults: The cardiovascular heart study. Presented at the American Heart Association's 41st annual conference on cardiovascular disease epidemiology and prevention. AHA. 2001.

Fenton WS, Dicerson F, Boronow J, et al. A placebo controlled trial of omega-3 fatty acid (ethyl eicosapentaenoic acid) supplementation for residual symptoms and cognitive impairment in schizophrenia. *Am J Psychiatry* . 2001;158(12):2071-2074.

Foulon T, Richard MJ, Payen N, et al. Effects of fish oil fatty acids on plasma lipids and lipoproteins and oxidant-antioxidant imbalance in healthy subjects. *Scan J Clin Lab Invest.* 1999;59(4):239-248.

Freeman VL, Meydani M, Yong S, Pyle J, Flanigan RC, Waters WB, Wojcik EM. Prostatic levels of fatty acids and the histopathology of localized prostate cancer. *J Urol.* 2000;164(6):2168-2172.

Friedberg CE, Janssen MJ, Heine RJ, Grobbee DE. Fish oil and glycemic control in diabetes: a meta-analysis. *Diabetes Care* . 1998;21:494-500.

Frieri G, Pimpo MT, Palombieri A, Melideo D, Marcheggiano A, Caprilli R, et al. Polyunsaturated fatty acid dietary supplementation: an adjuvant approach to treatment of Helicobacter pylori infection. *Nut Res* . 2000;20(7):907-916.

Gamez-Mez N, Higuera-Ciapara I, Calderon de la Barca AM, Vazquez-Moreno L, Noriega-Rodriquez J, Angulo-Guerrero O. Seasonal variation in the fatty acid composition and quality of sardine oil from Sardinops sagax caeruleus of the Gulf of California. *Lipids* . 1999;34)6_:639-642.

Geerling BJ, Badart-Smook A, van Deursen C, et al. Nutritional supplementation with N-3 fatty acids and antioxidants in patients iwth Crohn's disease in remission: effects on antioxidant status and fatty acid profile. *Inflamm Bowel Dis.* 2000;6(2):77-84.

Geerling BJ, Houwelingen AC, Badart-Smook A, Stockbrügger RW, Brummer R-JM. Fat intake and fatty acid profile in plasma phospholipids and adipose tissue in patients with Crohn's disease, compared with controls. *Am J Gastroenterol* . 1999;94(2):410-417.

Gibson SL, Gibson RG. The treatment of arthritis with a lipid extract of Perna canaliculus: a randomized trial. *Complement Ther Med* . 1998;6:122-126.

Griffini P, Fehres O, Klieverik L, et al. Dietary omega-3 polyunsaturated fatty acids promote colon carcinoma metastasis in rat liver. *Can Res* . 1998;58(15):3312-3319.

GISSI-Prevenzione Investigators. Dietary supplementation with n-3 polyunsaturated fatty acids and vitamin E after myocardial infarction: results of the GISSI-Prevenzione trial. *Lancet* . 1999;354:447-455

Halpern G-M. Anti-inflammatory effects of a stabilized lipid extract of *Perna canaliculus* (Lyprinol). *Allerg Immunol* (Paris). 2000;32(7):272-278.

Harper CR, Jacobson TA. The fats of life: the role of omega-3 fatty acids in the prevention of coronary heart disease. *Arch Intern Med* . 2001;161(18):2185-2192.

Harris WS. N-3 fatty acids and serum lipoproteins: human studies. *Am J Clin Nutr* . 1997;65(5):1645S (10).

Hayashi N, Tsuguhiko T, Yamamori H, et al. Effect of intravenous w-6 and w-3 fat emulsions on nitrogen retention and protein kinetics in burned rats. *Nutrition* . 1999;15(2):135-139.

Hibbeln JR. Fish consumption and major depression. *Lancet* . 1998;351(9110):1213.

Hibbeln JR, Salem N, Jr. Dietary polyunsaturated fatty acids and depression: when cholesterol does not satisfy. *Am J Clin Nut* . 1995;62(1):1-9.

Holman RT, Adams CE, Nelson RA, et al. Patients with anorexia nervosa demonstrate deficiencies of selected essential fatty acids, compensatory changes in nonessential

fatty acids and decreased fluidity of plasma lipids. *J Nutr.*
1995;125:901-907.

Homan van der Heide JJ, Bilo HJ, Tegzess AM, Donker AJ.
The effects of dietary supplementation with fish oil on renal
function in cyclosporine-treated renal transplant recipients.
Transplantation . 1990;49:523-527.

Horrobin DF. The membrane phospholipid hypothesis as a
biochemical basis for the neurodevelopmental concept of
schizophrenia. *Schizophr Res* . 1998;30(3):193-208.

Horrobin DF, Bennett CN. Depression and bipolar disorder:
relationships to impaired fatty acid and phospholipid
metabolism and to diabetes, cardiovascular disease,
immunological abnormalities, cancer, ageing and
osteoporosis. *Prostaglandins Leukot Essent Fatty Acids.*
1999;60(4):217-234.

Horrocks LA, Yeo YK. Health benefits of docosahexaenoic acid.
Pharmacol Res . 1999;40(3):211-225.

Howe PR. Can we recommend fish oil for hypertension? *Clin
Exp Pharmacol Physiol* . 1995;22(3):199-203.

Hrboticky N, Zimmer B, Weber PC. Alpha-Linolenic acid
reduces the lovastatin-induced rise in arachidonic acid and
elevates cellular and lipoprotein eicosapentaenoic and

126

docosahexaenoic acid levels in Hep G2 cells. *J Nutr Biochem* . 1996;7:465-471.

Hu FB, Stampfer MJ, Manson JE et al. Dietary intake of alpha-linolenic acid and risk of fatal ischemic heart disease among women. *Am J Clin Nutr* . 1999;69:890-897.

Iso H, Rexrode KM, Stampfer MJ, Manson JE, Colditz GA, Speizer FE et al. Intake of fish and omega-3 fatty acids and risk of stroke in women. *JAMA* . 2001;285(3):304-312.

Jeschke MG, Herndon DN, Ebener C, Barrow RE, Jauch KW. Nutritional intervention high in vitamins, protein, amino acids, and omega-3 fatty acids improves protein metabolism during the hypermetabolic state after thermal injury. *Arch Surg* . 2001;136:1301-1306.

Juhl A, Marniemi J, Huupponen R, Virtanen A, Rastas M, Ronnemaa T. Effects of diet and simvistatin on serum lipids, insulin, and antioxidants in hypercholesterolemic men; a randomized controlled trial. *JAMA* . 2002;2887(5):598-605.

Klurfeld DM, Bull AW. Fatty acids and colon cancer in experimental models. *Am J Clin Nut.* 1997;66(6 Suppl):1530S-1538S.

Kooijmans-Coutinho MF, Rischen-Vos J, Hermans J, Arndt JW, van der Woude FJ. Dietary fish oil in renal transplant recipients treated with cyclosporin-A: no beneficial effects shown. *J Am Soc Nephrol* . 1996;7(3):513-518.

Krauss RM, Eckel RH, Howard B, et al. AHA Scientific Statement: AHA Dietary guidelines Revision 2000: A statement for healthcare professionals from the nutrition committee of the American Heart Association. *Circulation* . 2000;102(18):2284-2299.

Kremer JM. N-3 fatty acid supplements in rheumatoid arthritis. *Am J Clin Nutr* . 2000;(suppl 1):349S-351S.

Kris-Etherton P, Eckel RH, Howard BV, St. Jeor S, Bazzare TL. AHA Science Advisory: Lyon Diet Heart Study. Benefits of a Mediterranean-style, National Cholesterol Education Program/American Heart Association Step I Dietary Pattern on Cardiovascular Disease. *Circulation* . 2001;103:1823.

Kris-Etherton PM, Taylor DS, Yu-Poth S, et al. Polyunsaturated fatty acids in the food chain in the United States. *Am J Clin Nutr* . 2000;71(1 Suppl):179S-188S.

Kruger MC, Coetzer H, de Winter R, Gericke G, van Papendorp DH. Calcium, gamma-linolenic acid and eicosapentaenoic acid supplementation in senile osteoporosis. *Aging Clin Exp Res.* 1998;10:385-394.

Kruger MC, Horrobin DF. Calcium metabolism, osteoporosis and essential fatty acids: a review. *Prog Lipid Res* . 1997;36:131-151.

Kulkarni PS, Srinivasan BD. Cyclooxygenase and lipoxygenase pathways in anterior uvea and conjunctiva. *Prog Clin Biol Res* . 1989;312:39-52.

Kuroki F, Iida M, Matsumoto T, Aoyagi K, Kanamoto K, Fujishima M. Serum n3 polyunsaturated fatty acids are depleted in Crohn's disease. *Dig Dis Sci.* 1997;42(6):1137-1141.

Laugharne JD, Mellor JE, Peet M. Fatty acids and schizophrenia. *Lipids* . 1996;31(Suppl):S-163-165.

Levy E, Rizwan Y, Thibault L, et al. Altered lipid profile, lipoprotein composition, and oxidant and antioxidant status in pediatric Crohn disease. *Am J Clin Nutr* . 2000;71:807-815.

Lockwood K, Moesgaard S, Hanioka T, Folkers K. Apparent partial remission of breast cancer in 'high risk' patients supplemented with nutritional antioxidants, essential fatty acids, and coenzyme Q10. *Mol Aspects Med* . 1994;15Suppl:s231-s240.

Lopez-Miranda J, Gomez P, Castro P, et al. Mediterranean diet improves low density lipoproteins' susceptibility to oxidative modifications. *Med Clin* (Barc) [in Spanish]. 2000;115(10):361-365.

Lorenz-Meyer H, Bauer P, Nicolay C, Schulz B, Purrmann J, Fleig WE, et al. Omega-3 fatty acids and low carbohydrate diet for maintenance of remission in Crohn's disease. A randomized controlled multicenter trial. Study Group Members (German Crohn's Disease Study Group). *Scan J Gastroenterol* . 1996;31(8):778-785.

Mabile L, Piolot A, Boulet L, Fortin LJ, Doyle N, Rodriquez C, et al. Moderate intake of omega-3 fatty acids is associated with stable erythrocyte resistance to oxidative stress in hypertriglyceridemic subjects. *Am J Clin Nutr* . 2001;7494):449-456.

Mayser P, Mrowietz U, Arenberger P, Bartak P, Buchvald J, Christophers E, et al. Omega-3 fatty acid-based lipid infusion in patients with chronic plaque psoriasis: results of a double-blind, randomized, placebo controlled, multicenter trial. *J Am Acad Dermatol* . 1998;38(4):539-547.

Meydani M. Omega-3 fatty acids alter soluble markers of endothelial function in coronary heart disease patients. *Nutr Rev* . 2000;58(2 pt 1):56-59.

Mitchell EA, Aman MG, Turbott SH, Manku M. Clinical characteristics and serum essential fatty acid levels in hyperactive children. *Clin Pediatr* (Phila). 1987;26:406-411.

Montori V, Farmer A, Wollan PC, Dinneen SF. Fish oil supplementation in type 2 diabetes: a quantitative systematic review. *Diabetes Care* . 2000;23:1407-1415.

Mori TA, Bao, DQ, Burke V, et al. Dietary fish as a major component of a weight-loss diet: effect on serum lipids, glucose, and insulin metabolism in overweight hypertensive subjects. *Am J Clin Nutr* . 1999;70:817-825.

Morris MC, Sacks F, Rosner B. Does fish oil lower blood pressure? A meta-analysis of controlled trials. *Circulation* . 1993;88:523-533.

Nagakura T, Matsuda S, Shichijyo K, Sugimoto H, Hata K. Dietary supplementation with fish oil rich in omega-3 polyunsaturated fatty acids in children with bronchial asthma. *Eur Resp J.* 2000;16(5):861-865.

Nestel PJ, Pomeroy SE, Sasahara T, et al. Arterial compliance in obese subjects is improved with dietary plant n-3 fatty acid from flaxseed oil despite increased LDL oxidizability. *Arterioscler Thromb Vasc Biol* . July 1997;17(6):1163-1170.

Newcomer LM, King IB, Wicklund KG, Stanford JL. The association of fatty acids with prostate cancer risk. *Prostate* . 2001;47(4):262-268.

Okamoto M, Misunobu F, Ashida K, et al. Effects of dietary supplementation with n-3 fatty acids compared with n-6 fatty acids on bronchial asthma. *Int Med* . 2000;39(2):107-111.

Okamoto M, Misunobu F, Ashida K, et al. Effects of perilla seed oil supplementation on leukotriene generation by leucocytes in patients with asthma associated with lipometabolism. *Int Arch Allergy Immunol* . 2000;122(2):137-142.

Olsen SF, Secher NJ. Low consumption of seafood in early pregnancy as a risk factor for preterm delivery: prospective cohort study. *BMJ* . 2002;324(7335): 447-451.

Prisco D, Paniccia R, Bandinelli B, et al. Effect of medium term supplementation with a moderate dose of n-3 polyunsaturated fatty acid on blood pressure in mild hypertensive patients. *Thromb Res*. 1998;91:105-112.

Paul KP, Leichsenring M, Pfisterer M, Mayatepek E, Wagner D, Domann M, et al. Influence of n-6 and n-3 polyunsaturated fatty acids on the resistance to experimental tuberculosis. *Metabolism* . 1997;46(6):619-624.

Peet M, Laugharne JD, Mellor J, et al. Essential fatty acid deficiency in erythrocyte membranes from chronic schizophrenic patients, and the clinical effects of dietary supplementation. *Prostaglandins Leukot Essent Fatty Acids* . 1996;55(1-2):71-75.

Puri B, Richardson AJ, Horrobin DF, et al. Eicosapentaenoic acid treatment in schizophrenia associated with symptom remission, normalisation of blood fatty acids, reduced neuronal membrane phospholipid turnover and structural brain changes. *Int J Clin Pract* . 2000;54(1):57-63.

Rhodes LE, Durham BH, Fraser WD, Friedmann PS. Dietary fish oil reduces basal and ultraviolet B-generated PGE2 levels in skin and increases the threshold to provocation of polymorphic light eruption. *J Invest Dermatol.* 1995;105(4):532-535.

Rhodes LE, White SI. Dietary fish oil as a photoprotective agent in hydroa vacciniforme. *Br J Dermatol.* 1998;138(1):173-178.

Richardson AJ, Puri BK. The potential role of fatty acids in attention-deficit/hyperactivity disorder. *Prostaglandins Leukot Essent Fatty Acids.* 2000;63(1/2):79-87.

Rose DP, Connolly JM, Coleman M. Effect of omega-3 fatty acids on the progression of metastases after the surgical excision of human breast cancer cell solid tumors growing in nude mice . *Clin Cancer Res* . 1996;2:1751-1756.

Sakaguchi K, Morita I, Murota S. Eicosapentaenoic acid inhibits bone loss due to ovariectomy in rats. *Prostaglandins Leukot Essent Fatty Acids* . 1994;50:81-84.

Sanders TA, Hinds A. The influence of a fish oil high in docosahexaenoic acid on plasma lipoprotein and vitamin E concentrations and haemostatic function in healthy male volunteers. *Br J Nutr* . 1992;68(1):163-173.

Seddon JM, Rosner B, Sperduto RD, Yannuzzi L, Haller JA, Blair NP, Willett W. Dietary fat and risk for advanced age-related macular degeneration. *Arch Opthalmol* . 2001;119(8):1191-1199.

Shils ME, Olson JA, Shike M, Ross AC. *Modern Nutrition in Health and Disease* . 9th ed. Baltimore, Md: Williams & Wilkins; 1999:90-92, 1377-1378.

Shoda R, Matsueda K, Yamato S, Umeda N. Therapeutic efficacy of N-3 polyunsaturated fatty acid in experimental Crohn's disease. *J Gastroenterol* . 1995;30(Suppl 8):98-101.

Simopoulos AP. Essential fatty acids in health and chronic disease. *Am J Clin Nutr* . 1999;70(30 Suppl):560S-569S.

Simopoulos AP. Human requirement for N-3 polyunsaturated fatty acids. *Poult Sci* . 2000;79(7):961-970.

Smith W, Mitchell P, Leeder SR. Dietary fat and fish intake and age-related maculopathy. *Arch Opthamol* . 2000;118(3):401-404.

Soyland E, Funk J, Rajka G, Sandberg M, Thune P, Ruistad L, et al. Effect of dietary supplementation with very-long chain n-3 fatty acids in patients with psoriasis. *N Engl J Med.* 1993;328(25):1812-1816.

Stampfer MJ, Hu FB, Manson JE, Rimm EB, Willett WC. Primary prevention of coronary heart disease in women through diet and lifestyle. *N Engl J Med* . 2000;343(1):16-22

Stark KD, Park EJ, Maines VA, et al. Effect of fish-oil concentrate on serum lipids in postmenopausal women receiving and not receiving hormone replacement therapy in a placebo-controlled, double blind trial. *Am J Clin Nutr* . 2000;72:389-394.

Stevens LJ, Zentall SS, Abate ML, Kuczek T, Burgess JR. Omega-3 fatty acids in boys with behavior, learning and health problems. *Physiol Behav* . 1996;59(4/5):915-920.

Stevens LJ, Zentall SS, Deck JL, et al. Essential fatty acid metabolism in boys with attention-deficit hyperactivity disorder. *Am J Clin Nutr* . 1995;62:761-768.

Stoll AL, Severus WE, Freeman MP, et al. Omega 3 fatty acids in bipolar disorder: a preliminary double-blind placebo-controlled trial. *Arch Gen Psychiatry* . 1999:56(5):407-412.

Stoll BA. Breast cancer and the Western diet: role of fatty acids and antioxidant vitamins. *Eur J Cancer* . 1998;34(12):1852-1856.

Terry P, Lichtenstein P, Feychting M, Ahlbom A, Wolk A. Fatty fish consumption and risk of prostate cancer. *Lancet* . 2001;357(9270):1764-1766.

Tsai W-S, Nagawa H, Kaizaki S, Tsuruo T, Muto T. Inhibitory effects of n-3 polyunsaturated fatty acids on sigmoid colon cancer transformants. *J Gastroenterol* . 1998;33:206-212.

Tsujikawa T, Satoh J, Uda K, Ihara T, Okamoto T, Araki Y, et al. Clinical importance of n-3 fatty acid-rich diet and nutritional education for the maintenance of remission in Crohn's disease. *J Gastroenterol* . 2000;35(2):99-104.

Ventura HO, Milani RV, Lavie CJ, Smart FW, Stapleton DD, Toups TS, Price HL. Cyclosporine induced hypertension. Efficacy of omega-3 fatty acids in patients after cardiac transplantation. *Circulation* . 1993;88(5 Pt 2):II281-II285.

von Schacky C, Angere P, Kothny W, Theisen K, Mudra H. The effect of dietary omega-3 fatty acids on coronary atherosclerosis: a randomized, double-blind, placebo-controlled trial. *Ann Intern Med* . 1999;130:554-562.

Voskuil DW, Feskens EJM, Katan MB, Kromhout D. Intake and sources of alpha-linolenic acid in Dutch elderly men. *Euro J Clin Nutr* . 1996;50(12):784-787.

Wagner W, Nootbaar-Wagner U. Prophylactic treatment of migraine with gamma-linolenic and alpha-linolenic acids. *Cephalalgia* . 1997;17(2):127-130.

Werbach MR. *Nutritional Influences on Illness* . 2nd ed. Tarzana, Calif: Third Line Press; 1993:13-22, 655-671.

Yehuda S, Rabinovitz S, Carasso RL, Mostofsky DI. Fatty acids and brain peptides. *Peptides* . 1998;19(2):407-419.

Yosefy C, Viskoper JR, Laszt A, Priluk R, Guita E, Varon D, et al. The effect of fish oil on hypertension, plasma lipids and hemostasis in hypertensive, obese, dyslipidemic patients with and without diabetes mellitus. *Prostaglandins Leukot Essent Fatty Acids* . 1999;61(2):83-87.

Zambón D, Sabate J, Munoz S, et al. Substituting walnuts for monounsaturated fat improves the serum lipid profile of hypercholesterolemic men and women. *Ann Intern Med.* 2000;132:538-546.

Zimmerman R, Radhakrishnan J, Valeri A, Appel G. Advances in the treatment of lupus nephritis. *Ann Rev Med* . 2001;52:63-78.

- Review Date: 5/1/2007
- Reviewed By: Participants in the review process include: Ruth DeBusk, RD, PhD, Editor, Nutrition in Complementary Care, Tallahassee, FL; Jacqueline A. Hart, MD, Department of Internal Medicine, Newton-Wellesley Hospital, Harvard University and Senior Medical Editor Integrative Medicine, Boston, MA; Gary Kracoff, RPh (Pediatric Dosing section February 2001), Johnson Drugs, Natick, Ma; Steven Ottariono, RPh (Pediatric Dosing section February 2001), Veteran's Administrative Hospital, Londonderry, NH. All interaction sections have also been reviewed by a team of experts including Joseph Lamb, MD (July 2000), The Integrative Medicine Works, Alexandria, VA;Enrico Liva, ND, RPh (August 2000), Vital Nutrients, Middletown, CT; Brian T Sanderoff, PD, BS in Pharmacy (March 2000), Clinical Assistant Professor, University of Maryland School of Pharmacy; President, Your Prescription for Health, Owings Mills, MD; Ira Zunin, MD, MPH, MBA (July 2000), President and Chairman, Hawaii State Consortium for Integrative Medicine, Honolulu, HI.
- Jordan, H, Matthan N, Chung M, Balk E, Chew P, Kupelnick B, DeVine D, Lawrence A, Lichtenstein A, Lau J. Effects of Omega-3 Fatty Acids on Arrhythmogenic Mechanisms in Animal and Isolated Organ/Cell Culture Studies. Evidence Report/Technology Assessment No. 92 (Prepared by Tufts-New England Medical Center Evidence-based Practice Center under Contract No. 290-02-0022). AHRQ Publication No 04-E011-2. Rockville, MD: Agency for Healthcare Research and Quality. March 2004.

138

- Balk E, Chung M, Lichtenstein A, Chew P, Jupelnick B, Lawrence A, DeVine D, Lau J. Effects of Omega-3 Fatty Acids on Cardiovascular Risk Factors and Intermediate Markers of Cardiovascular Disease. Evidence Report/Technology Assessment No. 93 (Prepared by Tufts-New England Medical Center Evidence-based Practice Center under Contract No. 290-02-0022). AHRQ Publication No. 04-E010-2. Rockville, MD: Agency for Healthcare Research and Quality. March 2004.
- Wang C, Chung M, Lichtenstein A, Balk E, Kupelnick B,, DeVine D, Lawrence A, Lau J. Effects of Omega-3 Fatty Acids on Cardiovascular Disease. Evidence Report/Technology Assessment No. 94 (Prepared by Tufts-New England Medical Center Evidence-based Practice Center under Contract No. 290-02-0022). AHRQ Publication No. 04-E009-2. Rockville, MD: Agency for Healthcare Research and Quality. March 2004.
- Schachter H., Reisman J, Tran K, Dales B, Kourad K, Barnes D, Sampson M, Morrison A, Gaboury I, and Blackman J. Health Effects of Omega-3 Fatty Acids on Asthma. Evidence Report/Technology Assessment No. 94 (Prepared by University of Ottawa Evidence-based Practice Center under Contract No. 290-02-0021). AHRQ Publication No. 04-E013-2. Rockville, MD: Agency for Healthcare Research and Quality. March 2004.
- MacLean CH, Mojica WA, Morton SC, Pencharz J, Hasenfeld Garland R, Tu W, Newberry SJ, Jungvig LK, Grossman J, Khanna P, Rhodes S, Shekelle P. Effects of Omega-3 Fatty Acids on Lipids and Glycemic Control in Type II Diabetes and the Metabolic Syndrome and on Inflammatory Bowel Disease, Rheumatoid Arthritis, Renal Disease, Systemic Lupus Erythematosus, and Osteoporosis. Evidence Report/Technology Assessment No. 89 (Prepared by Southern California/RAND Evidence-

based Practice Center under Contract No. 290-02-0003). AHRQ Publication No. 04-E012-2. Rockville, MD: Agency for Healthcare Research and Quality. March 2004.

- MacLean CH, Issa AM, Newberry SJ, Mojica WA, Morton SC, Garland RH, Hilton LG, Traina SB, Shekelle PG. Effects of Omega-3 Fatty Acids on Cognitive Function with Aging, Dementia, and Neurological Diseases. Evidence Report/Technology Assessment No. 114 (Prepared by Southern California/RAND Evidence-based Practice Center under Contract No. 290-02-0003). AHRQ Publication No. 05-E011-2. Rockville, MD: Agency for Healthcare Research and Quality. February 2005.
- Bonis PA, Chung M, Tatsioni A, Sun Y, Kupelnick B, Lichtenstein A, Perrone R, Chew P, DeVine D, Lau J. Effects of Omega-3 Fatty Acid Supplementation on Organ Transplantation. Evidence Report/Technology Assessment No. 115 (Prepared by Tufts-New England Medical Center Evidence-based Practice Center under Contract No. 290-02-0022). AHRQ Publication No. 05-E012-2. Rockville, MD: Agency for Healthcare Research and Quality. February 2005.
- Amaranth information and products can be found at www.nuworldamaranth.com
- Chia by Wayne Coats and Ricardo Ayerza Jr.
- Cooking with Chia by Gloria Hoover

Disclaimer

Printed in the United States
134180LV00004B/148/P

9 780615 238456